Benign Childhood Focal Seizures and Related Epileptic Syndromes

C.P. Panayiotopoulos

Benign Childhood Focal Seizures and Related Epileptic Syndromes

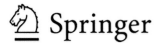 Springer

C.P. Panayiotopoulos MD, PhD, FRCP
Department of Clinical Neurophysiology and Epilepsies
St. Thomas Hospital
London SE1 7EH
United Kingdom
and
Department of Neurosciences
John Radcliffe Hospital
Oxford OX3 9DU
United Kingdom

ISBN 978-1-84996-476-0
Springer London Dordrecht Heidelberg New York

A catalogue record for this book is available from the British Library

Library of Congress Control Number: 2010936357

Cover design: eStudio Calamar S.L.

Printed on acid-free paper

Springer is part of Springer Science+Business Media (www.springer.com)

Contents

Preface

Over the last two decades, there have been spectacular advances in all fields of epilepsies. In clinical practice, the diagnosis of epilepsies has become more specific with the identification of epileptic syndromes and the treatment has expanded beyond the control of seizures to include improvement of quality of life.

Precise syndromic diagnosis, prognosis and management for every patient are the ultimate and often achievable goals. There is probably no better example than the benign childhood focal seizures and related epileptic syndromes to illustrate the significance of the specific diagnosis of epilepsies and the difference that this makes to patient and family.

Benign childhood focal seizures and related epileptic syndromes have a high prevalence probably affecting 22% of children with non-febrile seizures, are of excellent prognosis with remission by the age of 15 years or earlier, and constitute a significant part of the everyday practice of paediatricians, neurologists and electroencephalographers. They mainly comprise three identifiable electroclinical syndromes: rolandic epilepsy which is well known, Panayiotopoulos syndrome, a common autonomic epilepsy specific to childhood, which is currently more readily diagnosed and the idiopathic childhood occipital epilepsy of Gastaut, a less common form with uncertain prognosis. Neurological and mental states and brain imaging are normal, though because of their high prevalence any type of benign childhood focal seizures may incidentally occur in children with neurocognitive deficits or abnormal brain scans. The most useful diagnostic test is the EEG. In clinical practice, the combination of a normal child with infrequent seizures and an EEG showing disproportionately severe spike activity is highly suggestive of these benign childhood syndromes. However, some children may consistently have normal EEG.

Yet, despite significant progress in their clinico-EEG recognition, even for rolandic seizures expert opinions are still divided regarding genetics, neuropsychological consequences, management and relations to other syndromes of generalised and focal epilepsies. The situation is even less satisfactory for Panayiotopoulos syndrome, which despite sound clinico-EEG manifestations, is still widely misdiagnosed as encephalitis or other non-epileptic conditions, it is less well known amongst practising physicians though this is now unequivocally recognised by the new ILAE report which rightly abandoned the misleading descriptive terminology of "occipital epilepsy". The idiopathic childhood occipital epilepsy of Gastaut is often mistaken as a type of migraine though the visual aura of migraine is markedly different than the visual epileptic seizure.

With such a high prevalence and significance regarding prognosis, treatment strategies and psychosocial impact, the benign childhood focal seizures and related epileptic syndromes should be well understood and well known by those who care for the medical welfare of children such as paediatricians, paediatric neurologists, electroencephalographers and allied specialities. My enduring plea to the relevant official bodies is to re-examine the evidence and initiate research, scientific publications, practice parameter guidelines and public awareness campaigns as those that eliminated the myths and the anxiety regarding febrile seizures.

I hope that this concise booklet will serve to a better diagnosis and management of children with benign childhood focal seizures and related epileptic syndromes, which affect millions of children all over the world.

C P Panayiotopoulos MD, PhD, FRCP
June 2010
Oxford

Abbreviations

ADR	adverse drug reaction	ESES	extreme somatosensory evoked spike
AED	anti-epileptic drug		
APEC	atypical benign partial epilepsy of childhood	fMRI	functional magnetic resonance imaging
BCECTS	benign childhood epilepsy with centrotemporal spike	ICOE-G	idiopathic childhood occipital epilepsy of Gastaut
BCSSS	benign childhood seizure susceptibility syndrome	ILAE	International League Against Epilepsy
		MEG	magnetoencephalography
CAE	childhood absence epilepsy	MRI	magnetic resonance imaging
CT	computed tomography	MSA	multiple source analysis
CTS	centrotemporal spike	NREM	non-rapid eye movement
ECG	electocardiogram	PS	Panayiotopoulos syndrome
EEG	electroencephalogram	SGTCS	secondarily generalised tonic–clonic seizure

Introduction

Benign childhood focal seizures and related epileptic syndromes are the most common and probably the most fascinating and rewarding topic in paediatric epileptology.[1] They affect 25% of children with non-febrile seizures and form a significant part of the everyday practice of paediatricians, neurologists and clinical neurophysiologists who care for children with seizures. Rolandic seizures are widely recognised. Panayiotopoulos syndrome (PS), a previously unrecognised common disorder with dramatic clinical and EEG manifestations, has now been formally recognised by the ILAE.[2,3] It has further been highlighted by editorials[4,5] and reviews in medical journals,[6,7] examined in an expert consensus,[8] featured as the main theme of a recent issue of *Epilepsia*[7,9–12] and is becoming more readily diagnosed by physicians. Less common phenotypes, such as the idiopathic childhood occipital epilepsy of Gastaut (ICOE-G) and idiopathic photosensitive occipital lobe epilepsy, have also been recognised and defined. Furthermore, there are also children who present with seizures of predominantly affective symptoms, and claims have been made for other benign childhood seizures associated with certain inter-ictal *functional EEG foci*, such as frontal, midline or parietal, with or without extreme somatosensory evoked spikes (ESESs). All these conditions may be linked together in a broad, age-related and age-limited, benign childhood seizure susceptibility syndrome (BCSSS), which may also constitute a biological continuum with febrile seizures and benign neonatal and benign infantile seizures. BCSSS should be properly re-examined and redefined.

The term 'functional spikes' refers to transient focal EEG abnormalities of sharp waves that occur in children with or without epileptic seizures and which disappear in the late teens.[13]

Functional spikes of childhood are of low epileptogenic potential and they occur in 2% to 3% of normal children (Table).

EEG functional spikes in normal children (% median and range)			
Age (years)	Centrotemporal spikes	Occipital spikes	Frontal spikes	Generalised discharges
5–12	2.25 (0.7–3.5)	0.15 (0.0–0.4)	0.10 (0.1–0.6)	1.00 (0.1–1.1)
1–5	0.40 (0.3–0.4)	0.90 (0.8–1)	0.05 (0–0.1)	0.20 (0.1–0.3)

Modified with permission from Panayiotopoulos (1999).[1]

Considerations on classification

The ILAE Task Force recognises three syndromes of 'idiopathic childhood focal epilepsy':[2,3,189,190]

1. benign childhood epilepsy with centrotemporal spikes (BCECTS) (rating score 3)
2. Panayiotopoulos syndrome (3)
3. late-onset childhood occipital epilepsy (Gastaut type) (2).

The rating score in parenthesis reflects on the certainty with which the ILAE Core Group believed that each syndrome represents a unique diagnostic entity on a range of 1–3 (with 3 being the most clearly and reproducibly defined).[3] The 1989 ILAE classification recognised three 'age-related and localisation-related (focal, local, partial) epilepsies and syndromes':[189]

1. BCECTS
2. childhood epilepsy with occipital paroxysms (which is now called 'late-onset childhood occipital epilepsy [Gastaut type]')
3. primary reading epilepsy.

'Reading epilepsy' is now rightly classified as a reflex epileptic syndrome.[189]

Considerations on classification and nomenclature are detailed in the individual description of each syndrome. Overall, benign childhood focal syndromes and their main representatives, BCECTS and PS, do not fulfil the diagnostic criteria of 'epilepsy' defined as 'chronic neurological condition characterised by recurrent epileptic seizures'.[14] BCECTS and PS are age limited (not 'chronic') and at least a third of patients have a single (not a 'recurrent') seizure. They should be classified among 'conditions with epileptic seizures that do not require a diagnosis of epilepsy', which is a new concept in the ILAE diagnostic scheme that incorporates 'febrile, benign neonatal, single seizures or isolated clusters of seizures and rarely repeated seizures (oligoepilepsy)' (Table 5.2).[2,3,189]

Benign Childhood Epilepsy with Centrotemporal Spikes

1

Synonyms: BCECTS, rolandic seizures, rolandic epilepsy.

BCECTS[1,15–22] is the most common manifestation of benign childhood seizure susceptibility syndrome (BCSSS).

Considerations on nomenclature

I use the terms 'BCECTS', 'rolandic seizures' and 'rolandic epilepsy' synonymously, although I prefer the term 'rolandic seizures' for the following reasons:
- the term 'rolandic seizures' has long been established and is better known than BCECTS among paediatricians
- most 'centrotemporal spikes' (CTSs) are rolandic spikes; they are rarely located in the temporal electrodes
- the word 'temporal' is misleading because children with this form of epilepsy do not have symptoms from the temporal lobes
- BCECTS may occur without CTSs and conversely CTSs may occur in children without seizures or other clinical phenotypes of BCSSS[23]
- similar clinical features may appear in patients with spikes in locations other than at centrotemporal sites.

Demographic data

Onset is from age 1 to 14 years; 75% start between 7 and 10 years (peak 8 or 9 years).[1,17] There is a 1.5 male predominance. Prevalence is around 15% in children aged 1–15 years with seizures. Incidence is 10–20 per 100,000 children aged 0–15 years.

Clinical manifestations

The cardinal features of rolandic seizures are infrequent, often single, focal seizures consisting of:
- unilateral facial sensorimotor symptoms (30% of patients)
- oropharyngolaryngeal manifestations (53% of patients)
- speech arrest (40% of patients)
- hypersalivation (30% of patients).[1]

Hemifacial sensorimotor seizures are often entirely localised in the lower lip or spread to the ipsilateral hand. Motor manifestations are sudden, continuous or bursts of clonic contractions, usually lasting from a few seconds to a minute.

Ipsilateral tonic deviation of the mouth is also common. Hemifacial sensory symptoms consist of numbness in the corner of the mouth.

   Hemifacial seizures are often associated with an inability to speak and hypersalivation:

> The left side of my mouth felt numb and started jerking and pulling to the left, and I could not speak to say what was happening to me.

Oropharyngolaryngeal ictal manifestations are unilateral sensorimotor symptoms inside the mouth. Numbness, and more commonly paraesthesias (tingling, prickling, freezing), are usually diffuse on one side or, exceptionally, may be highly localised even to one tooth. Motor oropharyngolaryngeal symptoms produce strange sounds, such as death rattle, gargling, grunting and guttural sounds, and combinations:

> In his sleep, he was making guttural noises, with his mouth pulled to the right, 'as if he was chewing his tongue'.

> We heard her making strange noises 'like roaring' and found her unresponsive, head raised from the pillow, eyes wide open, rivers of saliva coming out of her mouth, rigid.

Arrest of speech is a form of anarthria. The child is unable to utter a single intelligible word and attempts to communicate with gestures. There is no impairment of the cortical language mechanisms:

> My mouth opened and I could not speak. I wanted to say I cannot speak. At the same time, it was as if somebody was strangling me.

Hypersalivation is often associated with oropharyngolaryngeal or pure hemifacial seizures. Hypersalivation is not just frothing:

> Suddenly my mouth is full of saliva, it runs out like a river and I cannot speak.

Ictal syncope may occur, probably as a concurrent symptom of PS:[189]

> She lies there, unconscious with no movements, no convulsions, like a wax work, no life.

Consciousness and recollection are fully retained in more than half (58%) of rolandic seizures:

> I felt that air was forced into my mouth, I could not speak and I could not close my mouth. I could understand well everything said to me. Other times I feel that there is food in my mouth and there is also a lot of salivation. I cannot speak.

Secondarily generalised tonic–clonic seizures (GTCSs) are reported in around half of children with rolandic seizures. Primarily GTCSs are not part of the syndrome of rolandic seizures (ictal EEG recordings), although the new ILAE report makes the unverified comment that 'some patients with this condition may have primarily GTCS as well'.[3]

Rolandic seizures are usually brief, lasting for 1–3 min. Three-quarters of seizures occur during non-rapid eye movement (NREM) sleep, mainly at sleep onset or just before awakening.

Status epilepticus

Although rare, focal motor status or hemiconvulsive status epilepticus is more likely to occur than secondarily generalised convulsive status epilepticus, which is exceptional. Opercular status epilepticus usually occurs in atypical evolutions of BCECTS[24–29] or, exceptionally, it may be induced by carbamazepine or lamotrigine,[30,31] and may last for hours to months. It consists of continuous unilateral or bilateral contractions of the mouth, tongue or eyelids, positive or negative subtle perioral or other myoclonus, dysarthria, speech arrest, difficulties in swallowing, buccofacial apraxia and hypersalivation.[189] These are often associated with continuous spikes and waves on an EEG during slow-wave sleep.

Aetiology

BCECTS is genetically determined, although conventional genetic influences may be less important than other mechanisms, which need to be explored.[32] There is evidence of linkage with chromosome 15q14.[33]

Autosomal dominant inheritance with age-dependent penetrance has been reported for subjects with CTSs on an EEG, and not for the clinical syndrome of BCECTS (see review in Panayiotopoulos[1]).[34,35] A recently published study found that the CTS EEG trait in rolandic epilepsy maps to Elongator Protein Complex 4 of chromosome 11p13.[35]

Siblings or parents of patients with BCECTS may rarely have the same type of seizures or other phenotypes of BCSSS, such as PS.[189] Febrile seizures are common (10–20%) before rolandic seizures.

See also the unifying concept of benign childhood seizure susceptibility syndrome.[1,36, 189]

Diagnostic procedures

Apart from the EEG, all tests are normal.

Brain imaging is not needed for typical cases, although 15% of patients with rolandic seizures may have abnormal findings because of static or other brain diseases unrelated to the pathophysiology of BCECTS.[37,38]

The presence of brain lesions has no influence on the prognosis of rolandic seizures.[37]

Electroencephalography

Inter-ictal EEG: CTSs are the hallmark of BCECTS (Figures 1.1, 1.2 and 1.3). They are age-dependent, appearing at a peak age of 7–10 years, often persisting despite clinical remission and usually disappearing before the age of 16 years. Although called CTSs, these are mainly high-amplitude, sharp and slow-wave complexes localised in the C3–C4 (central; Figure 1.2) or C5–C6 (midway between central and temporal) electrodes.[39] CTSs may be unilateral, but are more often bilateral, independently right or left. They are abundant (4–20/min) and usually occur in clusters.

CTSs amplify during stages I–IV of sleep by a factor of two to five times without disturbing sleep organisation. After sleep, the most common form of activation of CTSs (10–20%) is somatosensory stimulation, mainly of the fingers and toes (Figure 1.1).[1,40–47] These are extreme (giant) somatosensory evoked spikes (ESESs), which correspond to mid- or long-latency somatosensory evoked potentials with peaks at 35–80 ms, depending on the height of the individual and location of the site of stimulation (Figure 1.1). ESESs persist during sleep and, like spontaneous CTSs, occur in children with or without seizures and disappear with age. They may be detected in EEGs with or without spontaneous CTSs or other functional spikes of childhood.

> ## Practical note
>
> ### Elicitating ESESs in clinical EEG practice
> In clinical EEG practice, asking the child to tap together the palmar surface of the tips of his or her fingers of both hands is an easy method of testing for ESESs. The child should be instructed to strike them with sufficient strength and at random intervals of varying frequency. This may elicit either bilateral or unilateral ESESs (Figure 1.1).

Rarely, children with rolandic seizures may have a normal EEG: the spikes may be very small or CTSs appear only during sleep stages (3–35%).[1] In serial EEGs, CTSs may appear right or left, infrequently or frequently, small or giant, and alone or with functional spikes in other locations. The reported prevalence of generalised discharges in rolandic seizures varies from as low as 0% to as high as 54%.[1] In my studies, generalised discharges occurred in about 4% of patients with rolandic seizures, and consisted of brief 1–3 s generalised bursts of 3–5 Hz slow waves, mixed with small spikes.[1] These brief generalised discharges are identical to those seen in PS (Figure 1.4).

Dipole and magnetoencephalography (MEG) studies show that the main negative spike component of CTSs can usually be modelled by a single and stable tangential dipole source along the rolandic region, with the negative pole maximum in the centrotemporal region and the positive pole maximum in the frontal regions.[48–51] The tangential dipole and the location of CTSs have been confirmed with MEG.[52,53] More recently, combined spike-related functional MRI (fMRI) and EEG multiple source analysis (MSA) were applied.[54] EEG MSA

Video-EEG of an 11-year-old girl with rolandic seizures who has been in remission since the age of 8 years

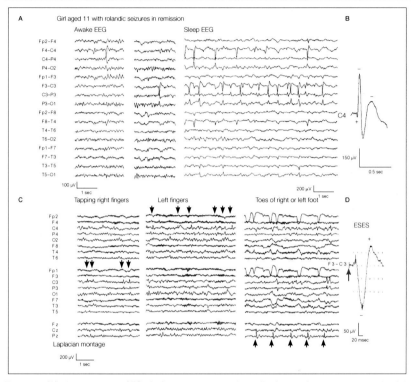

Figure 1.1 (**A**) High-amplitude CTSs (in fact, these are central spikes) occur independently on the right and left, and are markedly exaggerated during natural sleep. (**B**) Typical morphology and polarity of CTSs in laplacian montage. (**C**) ESESs, which are evoked by tapping fingers or toes. Note that their location corresponds to the location of the activating stimulus (black arrows). (**D**) ESES from another patient, which was evoked by electrical stimulation of the right thumb (onset at red arrow). Peak latency of the somatosensory evoked spike is 58 ms.

CTSs are mainly rolandic not temporal spikes[1,39]

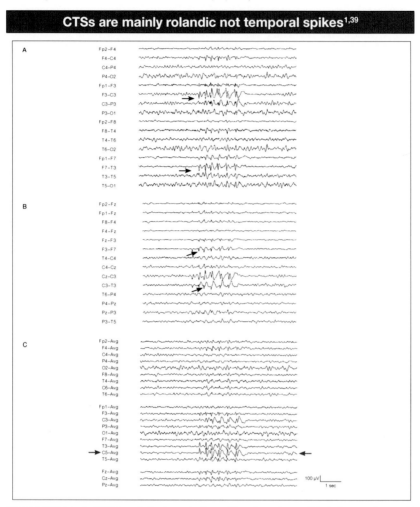

Figure 1.2 The same EEG sample is shown in three different montages. This is from an 8-year-old boy referred for an EEG because of: 'recent GTCSs and a 2-year history of unilateral facial spasms. Previously, the EEG and CT brain scan were normal. No medication. Focal seizures with secondarily generalised convulsions?' (**A,B**) The EEG showed frequent clusters of repetitive CTSs on the left. As the spikes appeared to be of higher amplitude in the temporal electrode (T3) (black arrows), the technician rightly applied additional electrodes at C5 and C6 (rolandic localisation) (**C**). This showed that the spike is of higher amplitude in the left rolandic region (C5) (red arrows). Another EEG 16 months later showed a few small spikes in the right frontal and central midline electrodes (not shown).

Video-EEG of a 10-year-old girl with rolandic seizures

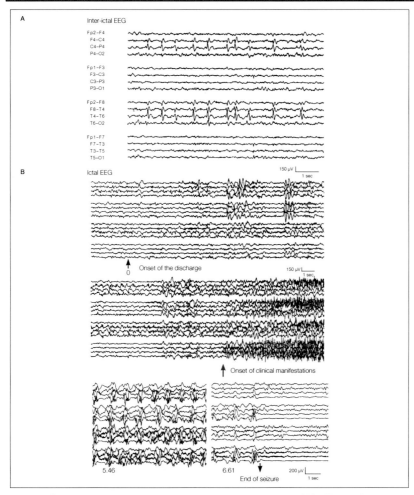

Figure 1.3 Case 5.1 in Panayiotopoulos.[1] (**A**) High-amplitude right-sided CTSs (C5 and C6 electrodes were not applied). (**B**) Onset of ictal discharge in the right centrotemporal regions during sleep (black arrow). Red arrow shows onset of clinical manifestations that started with contractions of the left facial muscles (note muscle artefacts on the left), progressing to a prolonged generalised clonic seizure, which lasted for 6.31 minutes from the ictal electrical onset. See video-EEG of this seizure in the companion CD of *A Practical Guide to Childhood Epilepsies*.[59]

confirmed the initial central dipole including the face or hand area. A second dipolar source was mostly consistent with propagated activity.[54]

> *The frequency, location and persistence of CTSs do not determine the clinical manifestations, severity and frequency of seizures or the prognosis.*
>
> *CTSs may also occur in normal children.*

It should be remembered that CTSs:
- occur in 2% to 3% of normal school-aged children, of whom less than 10% develop rolandic seizures (Table 1.1)[1,55–58]
- are common among relatives of children with rolandic seizures
- occur in a variety of organic brain diseases with or without seizures, such as cerebral tumours, Rett syndrome, fragile X syndrome and focal cortical dysplasia
- may incidentally be found in non-epileptic children with various symptoms, such as headache, speech, and behavioural and learning difficulties.

> *The combination of a normal child with infrequent seizures and an EEG showing disproportionately severe focal epileptogenic activity is highly suggestive of BCSSS.*[1]

Ictal EEG: There are very few reports of ictal EEGs of rolandic seizures. One example captured with video-EEG is shown in Figure 1.3. There is an initial paucity of spontaneous CTSs before the onset of the ictal discharge, which appears in the ipsilateral rolandic regions and consists of slow waves mixed with fast rhythms and spikes. This ended with a SGTCS.

Evolution and prognosis

The prognosis for rolandic seizures is invariably excellent, with a risk of developing infrequent generalised seizures in adult life of less than 2%; absence seizures may be more common than GTCSs.[1,60–63]

Remission occurs within 2–4 years of onset and before the age of 16 years. The total number of seizures is low, the majority of patients having fewer than ten seizures; 10–20% have just a single seizure. About 10–20% may have frequent seizures, but these also remit with age.

Children with rolandic seizures may develop reversible linguistic and cognitive abnormalities during the active phase of their disease.[1,64–66] Mainly hospital-based studies emphasise learning or behavioural problems that require intervention (see review by Nicolai, et al[67]).[66,68–73] However, the effect of anti-epileptic drugs (AEDs), bias in selection of the most serious cases and other factors were not taken into consideration in most of these studies (see the note of caution).

A few patients (<1%) may progress to atypical evolutions of more severe syndromes of linguistic, behavioural and neuropsychological deficits, such as

Landau–Kleffner syndrome, atypical benign partial epilepsy of childhood or epilepsy with continuous spike-and-wave during sleep.[27,28]

The development, social adaptation and occupations of adults with a previous history of rolandic seizures are normal.[1,62,63]

Note of caution

There is an increasing number of reports emphasising cognitive, linguistic and behavioural abnormalities of children with rolandic epilepsy. I am not in a position to dispute such findings. However, in most of these studies the findings are based on statistical comparisons of a group of children with rolandic epilepsy with matched normal control children. My reservations are that the groups of children with rolandic epilepsy include patients who are on AEDs, patients who may represent the worst spectrum of the disorder (i.e. hospital-based populations) or patients who have suffered bullying at school and social discrimination because of the stigma of 'epilepsy' with which they are often labelled. It is only if these factors are eliminated in studies of unbiased and newly diagnosed patients that we will learn of the true dimensions of the problem.[20]

Management

Children with rolandic seizures may not need AEDs, particularly if the seizures are infrequent, mild or nocturnal, or the onset is close to the natural age of remission of this age-limited disorder. Patients with either frequent seizures and secondarily GTCSs or comorbid conditions may need medication.[74] Some AEDs may significantly reduce GTCSs without reduction of focal seizures.[75] Empirically, carbamazepine is the preferred AED. Recent studies found levetiracetam to be highly effective.[76–78]

Some children might experience learning difficulties, aggravation and new types of seizures when receiving either carbamazepine[1,30,31,78,79] or lamotrigine.[80,81]

> Within days after re-introduction of carbamazepine, she suffered nearly continuous, brief atonic attacks of head and arm drop and also absences (case 17.3 in Panayiotopoulos[1]).

For details see 'Management of benign childhood focal seizures' on.[189]

Panayiotopoulos Syndrome

Panayiotopoulos syndrome (PS) is a common, childhood-related, idiopathic, benign susceptibility to focal, mainly autonomic seizures and autonomic status epilepticus.[4–12,20,23,82–101] Autonomic manifestations are the cardinal seizure symptoms in PS, and have immense pathophysiological, clinical and treatment implications, with all functions of the autonomic system possibly being affected during the ictus. Autonomic status epilepticus occurs in half of all patients.

A recent expert consensus defines PS as:

> A benign age-related focal seizure disorder occurring in early and mid-childhood. It is characterized by seizures, often prolonged, with predominantly autonomic symptoms, and by an EEG that shows shifting and/or multiple foci, often with occipital predominance.[8]

PS has been confirmed in long-term studies of over 1000 children worldwide. The importance of this syndrome and its impact on paediatric epileptology is signified by the June 2007 issue of *Epilepsia*, which featured PS as its main theme.[7,9–12]

Considerations on classification

PS has been initially recognised by the ILAE as 'early onset benign childhood occipital epilepsy (Panayiotopoulos type)'.[2,3] However, PS is not 'occipital' epilepsy:[7–11,20,90]

- onset is with autonomic manifestations, which are unlikely to be of occipital origin; of all the other seizure symptoms, only eye deviation, which is often not the first ictal symptom, may originate in the occipital lobes
- inter-ictal occipital spikes may never occur
- even ictal EEG has documented anterior or posterior origin.

Currently, most authors prefer the eponymous term 'Panayiotopoulos syndrome' to include all patients with this syndrome, irrespective of EEG spikes or topographical terminology,[4,5,23,90–94,97] as in the original study.[83] In this study, of the 21 children with ictal vomiting and normal neurological state evaluated,[83] 12 had occipital spikes 'epilepsy with occipital paroxysms'[98] and nine had extra-occipital spikes or normal EEG.[99]

In recognition of these unequivocal facts, the recent ILAE report retained only the eponymic "Panayiotopoulos syndrome" nomenclature and rightly abandoned the descriptive terminology of "occipital epilepsy".[190]

C.P. Panayiotopoulos, *Benign Childhood Focal Seizures and Related Epileptic Syndromes*,
© Springer-Verlag London Limited 2011

Demographic data

Onset is from age 1 to 14 years; 76% of cases start at 3–6 years of age (peak 4 or 5 years). Both sexes are equally affected.[90] Prevalence is around 13% in children aged 3–6 years with one or more non-febrile seizures, and 6% in the age group 1–15 years. In the general population, two to three of every 1000 children are affected. These figures may be higher if cases currently considered to have atypical features are included.[6,90]

Clinical manifestations

Seizures comprise an unusual constellation of autonomic, mainly emetic, symptoms, behavioural changes, unilateral deviation of the eyes and other more conventional ictal manifestations. Consciousness and speech, as a rule, are preserved at seizure onset. The seizure commonly starts with autonomic manifestations (81%), which are mainly emetic (72%). In a typical presentation, the child is fully conscious, able to speak and understand, but is complaining of feeling sick and looks pale:

> He complained of nausea and he looked pale. Five minutes later he vomited while still standing… He gradually became disorientated, but was still able to walk. However, 10 minutes from onset his eyes turned to the right and he became unresponsive.

Ictus emeticus: The full emetic triad (nausea, retching, vomiting) culminates in vomiting in 74% of seizures; in others, only nausea or retching occurs and, in a few cases, emesis may not be apparent. Emesis is usually the first apparent ictal symptom, but it may also occur long after the onset of other manifestations.

The initial manifestations do not suggest an epileptic seizure, as the child simply complains of feeling sick and being unwell, and vomits:

> On returning home from school, she looked tired and had a nap. After half an hour, she woke up looking pale and complained of feeling sick. She ran to the toilet and vomited repeatedly. Then her eyes deviated to one side and she became unresponsive and flaccid for 10 minutes. Soon after, she started recovering, answering simple questions and by 1 hour later she was playing again as if nothing had happened.

Autonomic manifestations other than ictus emeticus may occur concurrently or appear later in the course of the ictus. These include pallor or, less often, flushing or cyanosis; mydriasis or, less often, miosis; cardiorespiratory and thermoregulatory alterations; coughing; urinary and/or faecal incontinence; and modifications of intestinal motility. Hypersalivation (probably a concurrent rolandic symptom) may occur. Headaches and, more often, cephalic auras may occur, particularly at onset. *Pallor* is one of the most common ictal manifestations. It occurs mainly at onset, usually with emetic symptoms. Pallor may be among the first symptoms with no apparent emesis.

Cyanosis is less common than pallor and occurs principally during the evolution of the seizures, often while the child is unresponsive.

Urinary and faecal incontinence occurs when consciousness is impaired before, or without, convulsions:

> He became unresponsive and incontinent of urine.

Mydriasis is sometimes so prominent that it may be reported spontaneously:

> Her pupils were as big as her eyes.

Miosis is rare and occurs with other severe autonomic manifestations while the child is unresponsive.

Hypersalivation is also rare in PS, which is in contrast to its common occurrence in rolandic seizures. Combined speech arrest and hypersalivation, as in rolandic seizures, is even rarer.

Cephalic auras, although rare, are of interest because they are considered to be autonomic manifestations and because they may cause diagnostic confusion with migraine if they are not properly evaluated. Cephalic auras commonly occur with other autonomic symptoms, mainly nausea and pallor, at seizure onset. Occasionally, the child may also complain of 'headache' but whether the complaint of 'headache' is a true perception of pain, discomfort or some odd sensation in the head is uncertain:

> 'Funny feeling in my head', 'warm sensation', 'pressure', 'headache'.

Coughing may occur as an initial ictal symptom either with or without ictus emeticus. It is described as 'strange coughing' or 'cough as if about to vomit'.

Thermoregulatory changes: Raised temperature may be subjectively or objectively documented during the seizure or immediately post-ictally. Whether this is a coincidental finding, a precipitating factor or an ictal abnormality is uncertain, as it could be any of these. However, pyrexia recorded immediately after seizure onset is probably an ictal autonomic manifestation.

Abnormalities of intestinal motility: Diarrhoea (3%) is occasionally reported during the progression of seizures.

Breathing and cardiac irregularities are rarely reported, but may be much more common in a mild form. Breathing changes before convulsions include descriptions of 'heavy, irregular, abnormal breathing' or 'brief cessation of breathing for a few seconds'. Tachycardia is a consistent finding, sometimes at the onset of ictal EEG (Figure 2.2).

Cardiorespiratory arrest is rare, probably occurring in 1 per 200 individuals with PS.[8,90,100]

Ictal syncope (or syncopal-like symptoms) is a common and important ictal feature of PS.[6,8,10,90] In at least a fifth of seizures, the child becomes 'completely unresponsive and flaccid like a rag doll' before convulsions. Two-fifths have no convulsions or occur in isolation with no other symptoms.

> While talking to her teacher, suddenly and without warning, she fell on the floor pale, flaccid and unresponsive for 2 minutes. She had a

completerecovery, but 10 minuteslatershecomplainedoffeelingsick, vomited repeatedly and again became unresponsive and flaccid with pupils widely dilated for 1 hour. She had an unremarkable recovery and was normal after a few hours' sleep.

She complained of 'dizziness' and then her eyes deviated to the left, she fell on the floor and she became totally flaccid and unresponsive for 5 minutes.

I proposed the descriptive term 'ictal syncope'[90,101] to describe this state, because 'unresponsiveness with loss of postural tone' is the defining clinical symptom of syncope.[102,103] However, 'syncopal-like symptoms' may be more appropriate.[104] *Ictal behavioural changes* usually consist of restlessness, agitation, terror and quietness, which appear at the onset of seizures, often together with emetic or other autonomic manifestations. These symptoms are similar to those occurring in 'benign childhood epilepsy with affective symptoms'.[189]

At age 9 years, on returning from school, he looked tired and pale. He said that his head was killing him, 'something that would cause me to be sick'. In 10 minutes, he started screaming and banging his head on the wall. Within the next 20 minutes, he gradually became disorientated and floppy 'like a rag doll'. He was staring.

Conventional seizure symptoms

In PS, pure autonomic seizures and pure autonomic status epilepticus occur in 10% of patients. They start and end solely with autonomic symptoms. In all other seizures, autonomic manifestations are followed by the conventional seizure symptoms listed below.

Impairment of consciousness: Although initially fully conscious, the child gradually or suddenly becomes confused and unresponsive. Impairment of consciousness may be mild or moderate, with the child retaining some ability to respond to verbal commands, but often talking out of context occurs. In diurnal seizures observed from the onset, cloudiness of consciousness usually starts after the appearance of autonomic and behavioural symptoms. Good awareness may be preserved throughout the ictus in about 6% of seizures.

Deviation of the eyes: Unilateral deviation of the eyes is common, but it seldom occurs at onset. This pursuit-like deviation of the eyes may be brief (minutes) or prolonged (hours), continuous or less frequently intermittent.

Deviation of the eyes may occur without vomiting in 10–20% of patients and, in some children, the eyes may be open wide and remain in the midline before other convulsions occur.

Other ictal symptoms are, in order of prevalence, speech arrest (8%), hemifacial spasms (6%), visual hallucinations (6%), oropharyngolaryngeal movements (3%), unilateral drooping of the mouth (3%), eyelid jerks (1%), myoclonic jerks (1%), and ictal nystagmus and automatisms (1%). These probably reflect the primary area of seizure discharge generation. The seizures may end with hemi-convulsions, often with jacksonian marching (19%) or secondarily generalised convulsions (21%).

Ictal visual symptoms, such as elementary visual hallucinations, illusions or blindness, occur after more typical seizure symptoms of PS.

Seizure variations: The same child may have seizures with either marked autonomic manifestations or inconspicuous or absent autonomic manifestations. Seizures with no autonomic manifestations are rare (7%) and occur in patients who may also have additional autonomic seizures.[90]

The clinical seizure manifestations are roughly the same, irrespective of EEG localisations, although there may be slightly fewer autonomic and slightly more focal motor features at onset in children with no occipital spikes.[90]

Duration of seizures and autonomic status epilepticus: Almost half (44%) of the seizures last for more than 30 min and can persist for many hours (mean about 2 hours), constituting autonomic status epilepticus. The rest of the seizures (56%) last from 1 to up to 30 min with a mean of 9 min. Lengthy seizures are equally common in sleep and wakefulness. Even after the most severe seizures and status, the patient is normal after a few hours of sleep. There is no record of residual neurological or mental abnormalities. The same child may have brief and lengthy seizures. Hemiconvulsive or convulsive status epilepticus is exceptional (4%).

Circadian distribution: Two-thirds of seizures start in sleep; the child may wake up with similar complaints while still conscious or else may be found vomiting, conscious, confused or unresponsive. The same child may suffer seizures while asleep or awake.

Precipitating factors: There are no apparent precipitating factors other than sleep. Fixation-off sensitivity is an EEG phenomenon that may not be clinically important. Many seizures have been witnessed while a child is travelling in a car, boat or aeroplane. There are two explanations for this: (1) the seizures are more likely to be witnessed during travelling; and (2) children are more vulnerable because travelling also precipitates motion sickness, to which children are particularly susceptible.

Aetiology

PS, similar to the rolandic seizures, is probably genetically determined. Usually, there is no family history of similar seizures, although siblings with PS or PS and rolandic epilepsy have been reported.[9,23,84,87,91] There is a high prevalence of febrile seizures (about 17%), and there may be a high incidence of abnormal birth deliveries, although these all need re-evaluation.[90] A mutation in the *SCN1A* gene was recently reported in two siblings[104] and in a single case of severe PS with many febrile precipitants of seizures.[105] However, no such mutations were found in another couple of siblings with typical PS and no febrile seizure precipitants (personal communication with J. Livingston). These data indicate that SCN1A mutations when found contribute to a more severe clinical phenotype of PS.

Pathophysiology

Autonomic symptoms of any type are often encountered in seizures, whether focal or generalised, in adults or children, and they are implicated in occurrences of sudden death.[106,107] However, autonomic seizures and autonomic status with ictus emeticus and ictal syncope, with the symptomatology and sequence detailed here, are specific in childhood.[101] This clinical picture does not occur in adults: only about 30 cases of ictal vomiting have been reported, and not in the same sequence as in children – adult patients usually have amnesia about the vomiting, which often occurs after the seizure has started with other symptoms.[107–110] An explanation for this is that children are vulnerable to emetic disturbances as exemplified by 'cyclic vomiting syndrome', a non-seizure disorder of unknown aetiology that is also specific to childhood.[111] Ictal syncope is even more difficult to explain.

Symptoms at the onset of seizures are important, because they indicate the possible location of the epileptic focus. However, autonomic and emetic disturbances are of uncertain value with regard to localisation in PS and may occur in seizures starting from the anterior or posterior regions. The localisation of ictal vomiting in adults (the non-dominant temporal lobe) does not appear to apply to children.

Clinical and EEG findings indicate that, in PS, there is a diffuse and multifocal cortical hyperexcitability, which is related to maturation. This diffuse epileptogenicity may be unequally distributed, predominating in one area, which is often posterior. The preferential involvement of emetic and other autonomic manifestations may be attributed to epileptic discharges triggering temporarily hyperexcitable low threshold central autonomic networks of vulnerable children.[90,101] In other words, it is likely that in these children a 'weak' epileptic electrical discharge (irrespective of localisation) activates, at its onset, susceptible autonomic centres to produce autonomic seizures and autonomic status epilepticus. This happens before the generation of clinical manifestations from brain regions that are topographically related to the ictal electrical discharge (occipital, frontal, central, parietal and less often temporal) with clinical seizure thresholds higher than those of the autonomic centres.[20]

Koutroumanidis has proposed a modern view that PS is an important electroclinical example of benign childhood system epilepsy.[7]

Diagnostic procedures

Neurological and mental states and MRI are normal. However, see below under *Brain imaging* section. The most useful laboratory test is the EEG (Figure 2.1).

The determinant of neurodiagnostic procedures is the state of the child at the time he or she first presents medically, as follows:[90]

1. The child has a typical brief or lengthy seizure of PS, but has fully recovered before arriving at the accident and emergency department (A&E) or

EEG variability in Panayiotopoulos syndrome

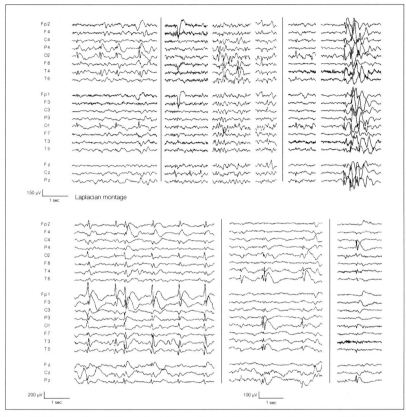

Figure 2.1 Samples from EEGs of six children with typical clinical manifestations of PS. Spikes may occur in all electrode locations, and they are usually of high amplitude and frequent or repetitive (clone-like repetitive multifocal spike–wave complexes), although they may also be small and sparse. Brief generalised discharges of small spikes and slow waves may be present.

being seen by a physician. A child with the distinctive clinical features of PS, particularly ictus emeticus and lengthy seizures, may not need any investigations other than an EEG. However, as about 10–20% of children with similar seizures may have brain pathology, MRI may be indicated.

2. The child with a typical lengthy seizure of PS has partially recovered, although he or she is still in a post-ictal stage, tired, mildly confused and drowsy on arrival at A&E or when seen by a physician. The child should be kept under medical supervision until full recovery, which, as a rule, occurs after a few hours of sleep. Then guidelines are the same as in (1).

3. The child is brought to A&E or is seen by a physician while ictal symptoms continue. This is the most difficult and challenging situation. Symptoms may dramatically accumulate in succession, and demand rigorous and experienced evaluation. A history of a previous similar seizure is reassuring and may help to avoid unnecessary investigation.

Electroencephalography

Inter-ictal EEG shows great variability. In about 90% of cases, the EEG reveals functional, mainly multifocal, high-amplitude, sharp–slow-wave complexes (Figure 2.1). Spikes may appear anywhere, often shifting from one region to another in a series of EEGs. Occipital spikes predominate but these do not occur in a third of patients. Spikes often appear independently in the same or the contralateral hemisphere. Clone-like, repetitive, multifocal spike–wave complexes may be characteristic features when they occur (19%).[90]

Small, and even inconspicuous, spikes may appear in the same or a previous EEG of children with giant spikes. Although rare, positive spikes or other unusual EEG spike configurations may occur.[90] Brief generalised discharges of slow waves, mixed with small spikes, may occur either alone (4%) or more often with focal spikes (15%).

Whatever their location, spikes are accentuated by sleep. EEG spikes may be stimulus sensitive; occipital paroxysms are commonly (47%) activated by the elimination of central vision and fixation,whereas CTSs may be elicited by somatosensory stimuli. Occipital photosensitivity is an exceptional finding.

The background EEG is usually normal, but diffuse or localised slow-wave abnormalities may also occur in at least one EEG in 20% of cases, particularly post-ictally.

EEG spikes may persist for many years after clinical remission or appear in only one of a series of EEGs.

A single routine EEG may be normal in 10% of patients. This should prompt a request for a sleep EEG.

The frequency, location and persistence of spikes do not determine clinical manifestations, duration, severity and frequency of seizures or prognosis. The clinical seizure manifestations are roughly the same irrespective of EEG spike localisation.

The multifocal nature of epileptogenicity in PS has been also documented with dipole analysis.[112,113]

Ictal EEG: Ictal video-EEG has unequivocally documented the epileptic nature of the autonomic manifestations in PS.[85,93,114-116] These may start long after the onset of the electrical ictal discharge and present as tachycardia, breathing irregularities, coughing or emesis, which would be impossible to consider as seizure events without an EEG. Other recognisable conventional seizure symptoms such as convulsions appear later in the ictal phase or may not appear at all. The seizure discharge mainly consists of rhythmic theta or delta activity, usually mixed with small spikes. Onset is unilateral, often posterior, but may also be anterior and not strictly localised to one electrode (Figures 2.2 and 2.3).

Magnetoencephalography

MEG revealed that the main epileptogenic areas in PS are along the parieto-occipital, calcarine or central (rolandic) sulci.[117,118] A more recent report of three children with PS (two were brothers) and frontal EEG spikes, showed equivalent current dipoles clustering in the frontal lobes (Figure 2.4).[119]

Brain imaging (Brain computed tomography scan and magnetic resonance imaging)

These by definition of an idiopathic epileptic syndrome are normal. However, considering the high prevalence of PS, coincidental brain abnormalities may be found and these do not appear to influence prognosis.[192,193]

Differential diagnosis

PS is easy to diagnose, because of the characteristic clustering of clinical seizure semiology, which is often supported by inter-ictal EEG findings. However, despite sound clinico-EEG manifestations, PS escaped recognition for many years and is still misdiagnosed for a number of reasons: [191]

- ictus emeticus was difficult to accept as a seizure event
- encephalitis or other acute cerebral insults were the prevailing diagnoses in the acute stage of a deteriorating level of consciousness followed by convulsions
- cardiogenic syncope, atypical migraine, gastroenteritis, motion sickness and a first seizure were the likely diagnoses when seizures were brief or after recovery from the acute stage.

Similarly, ictal syncope has only recently been recognised as an important clinical manifestation of PS; it may be misdiagnosed as cardiogenic syncope, pseudoseizure or a more severe encephalopathic state.[90]

The main problem is to recognise emetic and other autonomic manifestations as seizure events, and not to dismiss them or erroneously consider them as unrelated to the ictus and as a feature of encephalitis, migraine, syncope or gastroenteritis.

From a video-EEG of a 4-year-old boy with autonomic status epilepticus recorded from start to finish

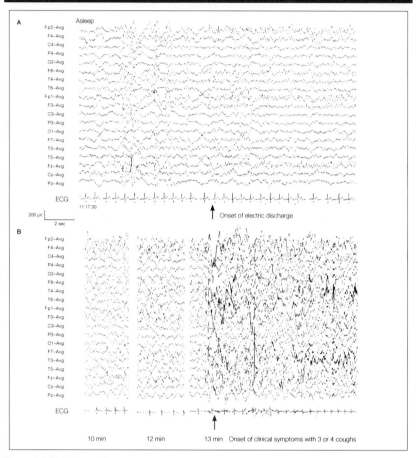

Figure 2.2 (A) High-amplitude spikes and slow waves are recorded from the bifrontal regions before the onset of the electrical discharge, which is also purely bifrontal (black arrow shows onset of ictal discharge). (B) First clinical symptoms with three or four coughs and marked tachycardia appeared 13 min after the onset of the electrical discharge (red arrow), when this had become bilaterally diffuse. Subsequent clinical symptoms were tachycardia, ictus emeticus (without vomiting) and impairment of consciousness. No other ictal manifestations occurred until termination of the seizure with diazepam 70 min after onset. Another lengthy autonomic seizure was recorded on video-EEG a year later. The onset of symptoms was different with mainly tachycardia and agitation.
Modified with permission from Koutroumanidis, et al (2005).[114]

Ictal EEG in Panayiotopoulos syndrome (A) and ICOE-G (B)

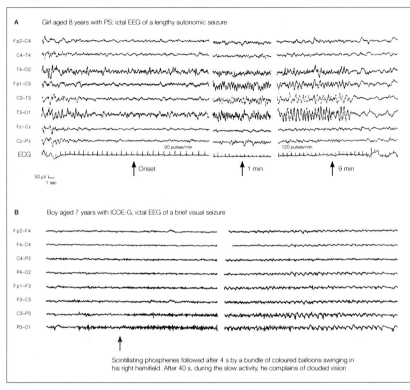

A   Girl aged 8 years with PS; ictal EEG of a lengthy autonomic seizure

Fp2–C4
C4–T4
T4–O2
Fp1–C3
C3–T3
T3–O1
Fz–Cz
Cz–Pz
ECG

90 pulses/min   120 pulses/min

↑ Onset   ↑ 1 min   ↑ 9 min

50 µV
1 sec

B   Boy aged 7 years with ICOE-G; ictal EEG of a brief visual seizure

Fp2–F4
F4–C4
C4–P2
P4–O2
Fp1–F3
F3–C3
C3–P3
P3–O1

↑

Scintillating phosphenes followed after 4 s by a bundle of coloured balloons swinging in his right hemifield. After 40 s, during the slow activity, he complains of clouded vision

Figure 2.3 (**A**) Samples of continuous EEG recordings from the onset to the end of a 9-min seizure during sleep stage II in an 8-year-old girl. Clinically, the seizure manifested with awakening, eyes opening, frequent vomiting efforts and complaints of frontal headache.[116] The ictal EEG started with remission of the inter-ictal occipital paroxysms and the appearance of occipital sharp rhythms progressing to monomorphic rhythmic theta activity in the bioccipital regions, mainly involving the right hemisphere in a wider posterior distribution. The slow activity slowed down with the progress of the seizure and ended with no post-ictal abnormalities. The ECG showed significant tachycardia during the ictus.[116] (**B**) Ictal EEG during a visual seizure in a boy with ICOE-G. The seizure starts in the left occipital region with fast spikes associated with visual symptoms. This spreads, 4 s later, to the parietal regions and the child sees a bundle of coloured balloons swinging in his right hemifield. This lasted for 40 s and was followed by slow waves that progressively became slower and diffused over the whole brain. At this stage, he complained of clouded vision. This boy was normal physically and intellectually, and also had a normal CT brain scan. At the age of 3 years, he had a nocturnal, left hemiconvulsion. His first EEG showed occipital paroxysms with fixation-off sensitivity. From the age of 4 years, he had started having frequent, brief, visual seizures (simple, coloured, visual hallucinations) provoked by sudden darkness.
Modified with permission from Beaumanoir (1993).[116]

MEG in Panayiotopoulos syndrome of frontal origin

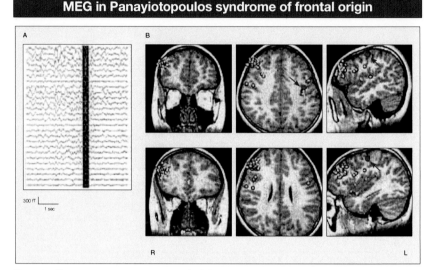

Figure 2.4 The patient had seizures typical of PS from the age of 4 years. EEGs initially showed occipital spikes, but at age 13 the EEG had bifrontal spikes and MEG was performed. His younger brother also had PS preceded by febrile seizures and followed by rolandic seizures. **(A)** MEG wave forms. The reversed coloured MEG wave forms in white in the vertical dark zone were analysed. **(B)** Magnetic source images revealed clustering equivalent current dipoles of spike discharges alongside the right inferior frontal sulcus, but the orientations were not so regular. All MRIs are T1-weighted. The pale-coloured solid circles and tails represent the locations and orientations of equivalent current dipoles of the spike discharges. The early somatosensory evoked field was modelled using a single equivalent current dipole approach to estimate the spatial source of response, whereas the dark-coloured solid circles and tails indicated by red arrows represent the locations and orientations of somatosensory evoked fields (N20). *Reproduced with permission from Saitoh, et al (2007).*[119]

It should be remembered that 10–20% of autonomic seizures and autonomic status epilepticus are due to heterogeneous cerebral pathology and are also restricted to childhood. These cases are betrayed by abnormal neurological or mental symptomatology, abnormal brain imaging and background EEG abnormalities.

PS is significantly different from rolandic seizures and ICOE-G despite some overlapping features.[20, 189] See also the unifying concept of benign childhood seizure susceptibility syndrome on page 41.[189]

PS should also be differentiated from febrile seizures, with which many of these children are diagnosed. However, febrile seizures are usually GTCSs from their onset. Conversely, GTCSs in PS occur only in a third of patients and happen after the onset of significant ictal autonomic manifestations (secondarily GTCS).

An EEG demonstrating multifocal spikes may be indispensable in the diagnosis of patients with PS if clinical information is inadequate or emetic manifestations are inconspicuous.

Prognosis

This syndrome is remarkably benign in terms of its evolution.[8,23,83–88,90–92,95,99,120,193] A quarter of patients with PS have a single seizure only and half have two to five seizures. The remaining quarter have more than six or sometimes very frequent seizures. Children with PS and neurobehavioral abnormalities may correlate with increased seizure burden in children with Panayiotopoulos syndrome.[120] Remission often occurs within 1 or 2 years of onset. Autonomic status epilepticus imparts no residual neurological deficit. Atypical evolution of PS with the development of absences, drop attacks and epilepsy with continuous spikes–waves during slow-wave sleep is extremely rare.[121,122]

A fifth of children with PS develop mainly rolandic seizures (13%) and less often occipital or other types of seizures during childhood and the early teens.[8,90,95] These are also age related and remit before the age of 16 years. The risk of epilepsy in adult life appears to be no higher than in the general population.[8,90]

Although the syndrome is benign in terms of its evolution, autonomic seizures are potentially life threatening in the rare context of cardiorespiratory arrest.[8,90,100] It is probably reassuring that normal children with epilepsy do not have an increased risk of death compared with the general population.[124]

Diagnostic tips

Paediatricians should be alerted by lengthy autonomic seizures, and electroencephalographers by frequent multifocal spikes in a normal child with one or a few seizures.

In terms of the EEG, it is important to remember that frequent epileptogenic foci in a normal child with infrequent seizures should raise the possibility of benign childhood focal seizures.

Management [6,8,10,20,90,101]

Current guidelines for febrile seizures, if appropriately modified, may provide the basis for similar guidelines for PS. Education about PS is the cornerstone of management. Prophylactic treatment with anti-epileptic medication may not be needed for most patients. Autonomic status epilepticus in the acute stage needs thorough evaluation; aggressive treatment may cause iatrogenic complications including cardiorespiratory arrest.

Idiopathic Childhood Occipital Epilepsy of Gastaut

Synonyms: ICOE-G, Gastaut-type of childhood occipital epilepsy, late-onset childhood occipital epilepsy (Gastaut type), childhood epilepsy with occipital paroxysms.

ICOE-G is a pure but rare form of idiopathic childhood occipital epilepsy.[1,20,95,125–129]

Considerations on classification

This purely 'idiopathic childhood occipital epilepsy' has been recognised in the new diagnostic scheme[2] as 'late-onset childhood occipital epilepsy (Gastaut type)' replacing the previous name 'childhood epilepsy with occipital paroxysms'.[130] Also note that 'benign' (used in all other benign childhood focal seizures) is not included in the descriptive terminology of this syndrome because ICOE-G is of uncertain prognosis.[2,130] Furthermore, the certainty by which the ILAE Core Group believed that this syndrome represents a unique diagnostic entity has been lowered to 2 on a score of 1–3 (3 being the most clearly and reproducibly defined).[3] My view is that ICOE-G is a definite but relatively rare epileptic syndrome of BCSSS.

The term 'idiopathic childhood occipital epilepsy of Gastaut' was chosen to (1) precisely describe that this is a purely occipital epilepsy, (2) honour this great epileptologist (Gastaut syndrome is an appropriate alternative but may be confused with Lennox–Gastaut syndrome) and (3) emphasise that there is no other type of idiopathic childhood occipital epilepsy.

Demographic data

Onset is between 3 and 15 years of age with a mean of around 8. Both sexes are equally affected. The disorder accounts for about 2–7% of benign childhood focal seizures.

Clinical manifestations

Seizures are purely occipital and primarily manifest with elementary visual hallucinations, blindness or both (see also the detailed symptomatology of occipital lobe epilepsy)[189]. They are usually frequent and diurnal, develop rapidly within seconds and are brief, lasting from a few seconds to 1–3 min, and, rarely, longer.

C.P. Panayiotopoulos, *Benign Childhood Focal Seizures and Related Epileptic Syndromes*, 27
© Springer-Verlag London Limited 2011

Elementary visual hallucinations as perceived and drawn by patients with visual seizures

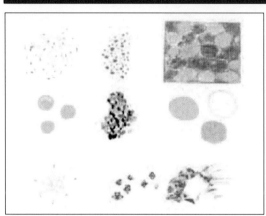

Figure 3.1 *Figure reproduced with permission from Panayiotopoulos (1999).*[1]

Elementary visual hallucinations are the most common and characteristic ictal symptoms, and are most likely to be the first and often the only clinical manifestation. They consist mainly of small multicoloured circular patterns (Figure 3.1) that often appear in the periphery of a visual field, becoming larger and multiplying during the course of the seizure, frequently moving horizontally towards the other side:[189]

> I see millions of small, very bright, mainly blue and green coloured, circular spots of light, which appear on the left side and sometimes move to the right.

Other occipital symptoms, such as sensory illusions of ocular movements and ocular pain, tonic deviation of the eyes, eyelid fluttering or repetitive eye closures, may occur at the onset of the seizures or appear after the elementary visual hallucinations.

Deviation of the eyes, often associated with ipsilateral turning of the head, is the most common (in about 70% of cases) non-visual ictal symptom. It is often associated with ipsilateral turning of the head and usually starts after visual hallucinations, although it may also occur while the hallucinations still persist. It may be mild, but more often it is severe and progresses to hemiconvulsions and GTCSs. Some children may have seizures of eye deviation from the start without visual hallucinations. It is likely that these cases have a better prognosis and shorter seizure lifespan than those with ICOE-G.[128]

Forced eyelid closure and eyelid blinking occur in about 10% of patients, usually at a stage at which consciousness is impaired. They signal an impending secondarily GTCS.

Ictal blindness, appearing from the start or, less commonly, after other manifestations of occipital seizures, usually lasts for 3–5 min. It can occur alone and be the only ictal event in patients who could, at other times, have visual hallucinations without blindness:

> Everything went suddenly black, I could not see and I had to ask other swimmers to show me the direction to the beach.[1,82]

Complex visual hallucinations, visual illusions and other symptoms resulting from more anterior ictal spreading rarely occur from the start. They may terminate in hemiconvulsions or generalised convulsions.

Ictal headache, or mainly orbital pain, may occur and often precedes visual or other ictal occipital symptoms in a small number of patients.[1,131]

Consciousness is not impaired during the visual symptoms (simple focal seizures), but may be disturbed or lost in the course of the seizure, usually before eye deviation or convulsions.

Ictal syncope is rare.[90]

Occipital seizures of ICOE-G may rarely progress to extra-occipital manifestations, such as hemiparaesthesia. Spread to produce symptoms of temporal lobe involvement is exceptional and may indicate a symptomatic cause.[1]

Post-ictal headache, mainly diffuse, but also severe, unilateral and pulsating, or indistinguishable from migraine headache, occurs in half the patients, in 10% of whom it may be associated with nausea and vomiting.

> I then have a left-sided severe throbbing headache for an hour or so.[1,131]

Circadian distribution: Visual seizures are predominantly diurnal and can occur at any time of the day. Longer seizures, with or without hemi or generalised convulsions, tend to occur either during sleep, causing the patient to wake up, or after awakening. Thus, some children may have numerous diurnal visual seizures and only a few seizures that are exclusively nocturnal or occur on awakening.

Frequency of seizures: If untreated, patients experience frequent and brief visual seizures (often several every day or weekly). However, propagation to other seizure manifestations, such as focal or generalised convulsions, is much less frequent (monthly, yearly or exceptionally).

Aetiology

There may be an increased family history of epilepsies (37% of cases) or migraine (16% of cases),[126] but a family history of similar seizures is exceptional.[132]

ICOE-G is considered to be a late-onset phenotype of BCSSS.[189]

Pathophysiology

The seizures are of a purely occipital lobe origin.[20,90]

The mechanisms for post-ictal headache, which is a common event after minor idiopathic or symptomatic visual seizures, with or without a predisposition to migraine, are unknown. It is likely that the occipital seizure discharge

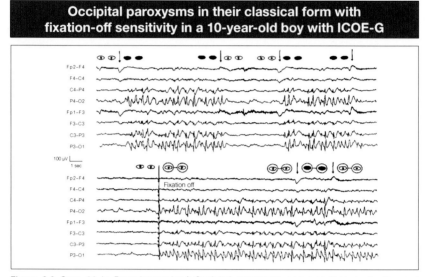

Occipital paroxysms in their classical form with fixation-off sensitivity in a 10-year-old boy with ICOE-G

Figure 3.2 Case 26 in Panayiotopoulos.[1] Occipital paroxysms occur as long as fixation and central vision are eliminated by any means (eyes closed, darkness, +10 spherical lenses, Ganzfeld stimulation). Under these conditions, eye opening cannot inhibit the spikes. Symbols of the eyes open or closed without glasses denote that the recording was made with the lights on and whenever fixation was possible. Symbols of the eyes open or closed with glasses denote that the recording was made when fixation and central vision were eliminated by any of the above means.
Reproduced with permission from Panayiotopoulos (1999).[1]

triggers a genuine migraine headache through trigeminovascular or brain-stem mechanisms.[131,133]

The occipital paroxysms are bilateral and synchronous when they occur, because they are activated in the bioccipital regions by the elimination of fixation and central vision (Figure 3.2).[90,134] They are not due to thalamocortical activation, as proposed by Gastaut and Zifkin.[126]

Diagnostic procedures

By definition, all tests other than the EEG are normal. However, high-resolution MRI is probably mandatory because of the high incidence of symptomatic occipital epilepsies with the same clinico-EEG manifestations.

Electroencephalography

The inter-ictal EEG shows occipital paroxysms, often demonstrating fixation-off sensitivity (Figure 3.2). However, some patients may only have random occipital spikes, whereas others may have occipital spikes only in the sleep EEG, and a few may have a consistently normal EEG. Centrotemporal, frontal and giant somatosensory evoked spikes may occur, although less often than in PS. Whether or not occipital photosensitivity is part of this syndrome is debatable.[189]

Occipital spikes are not pathognomonic of a particular syndrome, because they also occur in a variety of organic brain diseases with or without seizures, in children with congenital or early onset visual and ocular deficits, and even in 0.8–1% of normal preschool-age children (Table in introduction).[55,134–136] They are common in young children, with a peak age at first discovery of 4–5 years, and 'tend to disappear in adult life, and the subsidence of the EEG abnormality is usually accompanied by a cessation of seizures'.[55,135]

Ictal EEG, preceded by regression of occipital paroxysms, is characterised by the sudden appearance of an occipital discharge that consists of fast rhythms, fast spikes or both (Figure 2.3).[116,125,126,137–141] This is of a much lower amplitude than the inter-ictal occipital spikes. Elementary visual hallucinations are related to the fast-spike activity. Complex visual hallucinations may occur when the discharge is slower. In oculoclonic seizures, spikes and spikes and waves are slower, and a localised ictal fast spike rhythm may occur before deviation of the eyes. Ictal EEG during blindness is characterised by pseudo-periodic slow waves and spikes, which differ from those seen in ictal visual hallucinations.

There are usually no post-ictal abnormalities.

Differential diagnosis

The differential diagnosis of ICOE-G is mainly from cryptogenic or symptomatic occipital epilepsy, coeliac disease, migraine with aura, and basilar or acephalgic migraine where misdiagnosis is high.[1,131]

The differential diagnosis from migraine should be easy if all clinical elements are properly assessed and synthesised.[189]

Basilar migraine with occipital spikes does not exist; the relevant reports described cases with genuine ICOE-G imitating basilar migraine.[131,142,189]

Symptomatic occipital epilepsy often imitates ICOE-G; neuro-ophthalmological examination and brain imaging may be normal. Thus, high-resolution MRI is required to detect subtle lesions.

Occipital seizures of mitochondrial disorders, Lafora disease and coeliac disease[143] should be considered.[1,189]

Differentiating idiopathic childhood occipital epilepsy of Gastaut from Panayiotopoulos syndrome

The differentiation here is straightforward and statistically validated.[1] The seizures of ICOE-G are purely occipital and as such start and often end only with occipital lobe symptomatology. Further, seizures are mainly brief, frequent and diurnal. Rarely, seizures may be longer and also occur in sleep, but these are also fundamentally different to the rolandic epilepsy or the autonomic seizures and autonomic status epilepticus of PS (Table 3.1). Exceptionally, ictal vomiting may occur in ICOE-G but this follows the appearance of visual symptomatology, as occurs with reflex photosensitive occipital seizures, and the same patient usually has frequent brief occipital seizures. Conversely, visual symptoms in

Main features of rolandic epilepsy, Panayiotopoulos syndromes and idiopathic childhood occipital epilepsy of Gastaut

	Rolandic epilepsy	Panayiotopoulos syndrome	Idiopathic childhood occipital epilepsy of Gastaut
Febrile seizures (%)	18	17	10
Prognosis	Excellent	Excellent	Uncertain
Remission within 1–2 years from first seizure	Common	Common	Exceptional or rare
Seizures after the age of 13 years	Rare	Exceptional	Common
Interictal EEG			
Centrotemporal spikes alone	As a rule and characteristic	Rare	Have not been reported
Occipital spikes	Have not been reported	65%	Probably 90%
Spikes in other locations	Probably uncommon	Frequent	Exceptional
Brief generalised discharged of 3–5Hz slow waves with small spikes (%)	5	10	Exceptional
Somatosensory evoked spikes	Common	Rare	Have not been reported
Fixation-off sensitivity	Has not been reported	Rare	May be less common than reported
Photosensitivity	Has not been reported	Exceptional	Probably 20–30%
Normal EEG or focal slow after first seizure (%)	~10	~10	~10
Ictal EEG	Slow activity with spikes	Slow activity with spikes	Fast spikes and fast rhythms
Ictal onset	Rolandic regions	Anterior or posterior regions	Occipital regions
Prevalence amongst children aged 1–15 years	15	6	0.5–1with non-febrile seizures (%)
Peak age at onset (years)	7–10	3–6	8–11
Male to female ratio	1.5	1	1
Seizure characteristics			
Typical onset with	Hemifacial sensory-motor or oropharyngolaryn-geal symptoms	Autonomic symptoms mainly with emesis	Visual symptoms mainly with elementary visual hallucinations

Main features of rolandic epilepsy, Panayiotopoulos syndromes and idiopathic childhood occipital epilepsy of Gastaut

	Rolandic epilepsy	Panayiotopoulos syndrome	Idiopathic childhood occipital epilepsy of Gastaut
Hemifacial sensory-motor symptoms	Common and often from onset	Rare and not from onset	Rare and not from onset
Oropharyngolaryngeal symptoms	Common and often from onset	Rare and not from onset	Have not been reported
Speech arrest	Common and often from onset	Rare and not from onset	Has not been reported
Hypersalivation	Common and often from onset	Rare and not from onset	Has not been reported
Ictus emeticus	Rare and not from onset	Common and often from onset	Rare and not from onset
Autonomic disturbances other than vomiting and hypersalivation	Exceptional and not from onset	Common and often from onset	Exceptional and not from onset
Visual symptoms	Have not been reported	7% but exceptional from onset	Common and often from onset
Deviation of the eyes	Frequent during sensory-motor symptoms	Common but rarely from onset	Common but rarely from onset
Ictal behavioural changes	Exceptional and not from onset	Common and often from onset	Have not been reported
Duration for 1–3min	As a rule	Rare	As a rule
Duration of more than 5min	Rare	Common	Rare
Partial status epilepticus (>30min)	Exceptional	40%	Exceptional
Total number of seizures 1–15	As a rule	As a rule	Rare
Single seizures only (%)	10–20	30	Exceptional
Frequent seizures (%)	10	10	90
Nocturnal (sleep only) (%)	70	64	Exceptional

Table 3.1 *Continued from facing page.*
Reproduced with permission from Panayiotopoulos et al (2008).[20]

PS, when present, are not the sole manifestation of a seizure or stereotypical; only exceptionally (1%) are they reported at seizure onset.[9,84,90] From the EEG standpoint, the occipital spikes that characterise ICOE-G are also common in PS, but these often occur with extra-occipital spikes and with shifting locations in sequential EEG (Figure 2.1). Further, ictal EEG is markedly different between these syndromes (Figure 2.3). Some reported difficulties in differentiating ICOE-G from PS[144] may arise when emphasis is unduly placed on individual symptoms that may overlap, rather than on a comprehensive synthetic analysis of their quality, chronological sequence and other clustering features in the respective electro-clinical phenotypes, which is the basis for precise differential diagnosis in clinical practice. If any other diagnostic approach is followed, then even non-epileptic disorders such as migraine with aura could be deemed as overlapping with ICOE-G (visual hallucinations and headache), PS (lengthy duration and vomiting) or both (age, family history of epilepsies). It may be because of these limitations and the retrospective character of their study that Taylor et al. (2008)[144] found that only one of their 16 patients was typical in all respects of PS and that ICOE-G was as frequent as PS, which contrasts with all previous prospective studies cited in this chapter. Such a discrepancy may indicate that PS is still unrecognised even by epileptologists and that the study does not represent the vast majority of typical PS. Further, the commonly quoted argument that PS is not essentially different from ICOE-G, "considering that the younger the children are, the less likely they are to describe visual symptoms," is not tenable: (i) more than two-thirds of children with PS are older than 4 years and therefore able to describe their visual experiences and (ii) there is no difference in seizure presentation between younger and older children with PS. A few patients with either PS or rolandic epilepsy may later develop purely occipital seizures as of ICOE-G. These cases are easy to diagnose and indicate the intimate links of these disorders within the framework of BCSSS.[189]

Prognosis

The prognosis of ICOE-G is unclear, although available data indicate that re-mission occurs in 50–60% of patients within 2–4 years of onset. Seizures show a dramatically good response to carbamazepine in more than 90% of patients. However, 40–50% of patients may continue to have visual seizures and in-frequent secondarily GTCSs, particularly if they have not been appropriately treated with carbamazepine. Rarely, atypical evolutions to epilepsy with contin-uous spikes and waves during slow-wave sleep and cognitive deterioration have been reported.[145] Also rarely, children with ICOE-G may manifest with typical absence seizures, which usually appear after the onset of visual seizures.[146]

Although no significant differences were found in basic neurophysiological functions between patients with ICOE-G and control groups, patients' performance scores for attention, memory and intellectual functioning were lower.[147]

Management

In contrast to other phenotypes of the BCSSS, patients with ICOE-G often suffer from frequent seizures and therefore medical treatment, mainly with carbamazepine, is likely to be mandatory.[1,131] Secondarily GTCSs are probably unavoidable without medication.

A slow reduction in the dose of medication 2 or 3 years after the last visual or other minor or major seizure should be advised, but if visual seizures reappear, treatment should be restored. See details in the section on Management.[189]

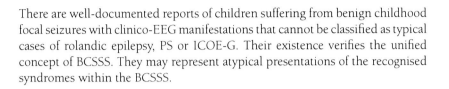

Other Phenotypes of Benign Childhood Focal Seizures[1]

There are well-documented reports of children suffering from benign childhood focal seizures with clinico-EEG manifestations that cannot be classified as typical cases of rolandic epilepsy, PS or ICOE-G. Their existence verifies the unified concept of BCSSS. They may represent atypical presentations of the recognised syndromes within the BCSSS.

Benign childhood seizures with affective symptoms

Benign childhood epilepsy with affective symptoms[29,148] is a rare clinical phenotype of the BCSSS with features common in both PS (behavioural and autonomic symptoms) and rolandic epilepsy (arrest of speech and hypersalivation).

Demographic data

Onset is between 2 and 9 years of age. Both sexes are equally affected. Prevalence may be very low.

Clinical manifestations

Seizures manifest with terror and screaming, autonomic disturbances (pallor, sweating, abdominal pain, salivation), chewing and other automatisms, mild impairment of consciousness and arrest of speech.

The predominant seizure symptom is sudden fear or terror:

> This terror was expressed by the child starting to scream, to yell or to call his mother; he clung to her or to anyone nearby or went to a corner of the room hiding his face in his hands. His terrorised expression was sometimes associated with either chewing or swallowing movements, distressed laughter, arrest of speech with glottal noises, moans and salivation, or some kind of autonomic manifestation, such as pallor, sweating or abdominal pain, that the child expressed by bringing his hands onto his abdomen and saying 'It hurts me, it hurts me'. These phenomena were associated with changes in awareness (loss of contact) that did not amount to complete unconsciousness.[148]

The seizures are brief, lasting between 1 and 2 min, with a maximum duration of 10 min.

C.P. Panayiotopoulos, *Benign Childhood Focal Seizures and Related Epileptic Syndromes*, 37
© Springer-Verlag London Limited 2011

Half the children have frequent (several times a day) seizures from the onset of the disease, which may occur with the same semiology, whether awake or asleep. Some children may have brief and infrequent nocturnal rolandic seizures at the same time as the affective attacks. Generalised seizures do not occur.

Aetiology

This is probably a rare phenotype of BCSSS or may be atypical presentations of PS and rolandic epilepsy.

A fifth of patients have febrile seizures, and a family history of undefined types of epilepsy are common (36%).

Diagnostic procedures

All tests, apart from the EEG, are normal.

Electroencephalography[29,148]

The inter-ictal EEG shows high-amplitude functional spikes located around the fronto- and parietotemporal electrodes. These are exaggerated by sleep and may be associated with generalised discharges.

Ictal EEG discharges are localised to the frontotemporal, centrotemporal or parietal areas, or may be diffuse. They are stereotypical in each individual patient.

Prognosis

Remission occurs within 1 or 2 years of onset. At the active stage of the disease, behavioural problems may be prominent, but subside with the seizures. The response to treatment is excellent.

Management

In the active phase of the disease and because of the frequent seizures, anti-epileptic medication, mainly carbamazepine, may be needed.

Benign childhood epilepsy with parietal spikes and frequent ESESs

Benign childhood epilepsy with parietal spikes and frequent ESESs[40,45,149] may be another phenotype of BCSSS. Defining features are EEG spikes in parietal regions, which are often elicited by tactile stimulation. However, ESESs[1,40–42,45,46,90,189] are not specific for any syndrome because they also occur in 10–20% of children with rolandic seizures (Figure 1.1),[45] in a few patients with PS[1,90] and in children with no seizures.[150]

Clinically, patients suffer from versive seizures of the head and body, often without impairment of consciousness. These are mainly diurnal and infrequent. Multiple daily seizures and focal status epilepticus are exceptional.

Remission usually occurs within 1 year of seizure onset, but EEG abnormalities may persist for longer.

Benign childhood focal seizures associated with frontal or midline spikes

Benign childhood focal seizures associated with frontal[1,151,152] or midline spikes[1,153] have been described and long follow-up reports have confirmed a benign course, although no systematic studies have been published. However, it should be remembered that EEG spike foci of various locations are also seen in rolandic epilepsy and more commonly in PS. Midline spikes are more common in children than in adults and they are not specific for any type of epilepsy.[154,155] Of six children with at least one EEG having only midline spikes, five had normal development with febrile seizures (one case), rolandic epilepsy (one case), PS (one case), a single complex focal occipital seizure (one case) or brief seizures with loss of consciousness only (one case). The only symptomatic case had generalised convulsions.[155]

Benign infantile focal epilepsy with midline spikes and waves during sleep

Benign infantile focal epilepsy with midline spikes and waves during sleep (or benign focal epilepsy in infants with central and vertex spikes and waves during sleep) has been recently described as a new BCSSS.[156–159] In terms of age, this is borderline between benign infantile seizures of Watanabe- Vigevano syndrome and BCSSS.[189] Age at onset is in the first 3 years of life and both sexes are equally affected. Infants are normal and all tests other than the EEG are normal. Seizures consist mainly of staring, motion arrest, facial cyanosis, loss of consciousness and stiffening of the arms. Clonic convulsions and automatisms are rare. Duration of seizures is from 1 to 5 min. Seizures are mainly diurnal (but may also occur during sleep), they may occur in clusters and are generally infrequent (one to three seizures per year). There is a strong family history of undefined types of epileptic seizures, with benign epilepsies prevailing.

Inter-ictal EEG abnormalities are seen only in NREM sleep and consist of small, mostly singular, midline spikes and waves.

The prognosis is excellent, with remission of seizures, normal development and normalisation of the EEG before the age of 4.

Benign Childhood Seizure Susceptibility Syndrome: A Unified Concept

5

Benign childhood focal seizures with focal EEG sharp–slow-wave complexes are probably a group of syndromes of one nosological continuum.[1,20,36,90] They share common clinical and EEG characteristics. Seizures are infrequent, usually nocturnal and remit within 1–3 years of onset. Brief or prolonged seizures, even status epilepticus, may be the only clinical event in the patient's lifetime. Ictal autonomic manifestations, such as hypersalivation, emesis, headache and ictal syncope, which are unusual in other epileptic syndromes or in adults, are frequent and may occasionally appear in isolation. The clinical and EEG characteristics of one syndrome may evolve into another or a child may simultaneously develop features of another form of benign childhood focal seizures.

Febrile seizures are common. Neurological and intellectual states are normal, but some children may experience mild and reversible neuropsychological problems during the active stage of the disorder. Brain imaging is normal. There are usually severe EEG abnormalities of spikes, which are disproportionate to the frequency of seizures. Epileptogenic foci, irrespective of their location, manifest as abundant, high-amplitude, sharp–slow-wave complexes which occur mainly in clusters. They are often bilateral, independent or synchronous, frequently combined with foci from other cortical areas or brief generalised discharges, and are exaggerated in sleep stages I–IV. A normal EEG is rare and should prompt a sleep EEG study. Similar EEG features, which resolve with age, are found in normal school-age children (Table in introduction) and 1% of children who have had an EEG for reasons other than seizures.

There is no justification for suggesting that all these syndromes differ merely because an 'epileptogenic' focus is a little anterior or posterior, or lateral or medial to the centrotemporal regions. A unified concept of benign childhood focal seizures is also suggested by the frequency of more than one type of benign childhood focal seizures in an affected child, siblings or both.

In all probability, all these conditions are linked together by a common, genetically determined, mild and reversible, functional derangement of the maturational process of the brain.[1,36] This derangement is often clinically silent and presents in more than 90% with EEG sharp and slow waves that are age related. The remaining minority have infrequent focal seizures with symptoms that are localisation and age related and dependent. A few of these children, with or without seizures, could also possibly have minor and fully

C.P. Panayiotopoulos, *Benign Childhood Focal Seizures and Related Epileptic Syndromes*, 41
© Springer-Verlag London Limited 2011

reversible neuropsychological symptoms that are rarely clinically overt and can be detected only by formal neuropsychological testing. Finally, there may be a very small number of patients (<1%) in whom this derangement of brain maturation may be further derailed to a more aggressive condition with seizures, neuropsychological manifestations and EEG abnormalities of various combinations and various degrees of severity, such as atypical benign focal epilepsy of childhood, Landau–Kleffner syndrome and epilepsy with continuous spike-and-slow-wave during sleep.[189]

My overall impression and appeal is that benign childhood focal seizures, and their clinical and EEG manifestations and evolutions, need appropriate prospective studies, such as those performed for febrile seizures.

Age-related childhood susceptibility to benign seizures

One of the most interesting aspects of benign childhood seizures is their striking age-related sequence. Benign neonatal and infantile seizures, febrile seizures, rolandic epilepsy, PS and other clinical phenotypes of BCSSS are specific to children and do not occur in adults. That children are particularly susceptible to seizures is well documented.

There are three main periods of age-related childhood susceptibility to benign seizures (Figure 5.1):

1. Febrile, mainly *generalised*, convulsions first appear in early childhood at a peak age of around 18–22 months.
2. PS covers the intermediate period, occurring at a peak of 4 or 5 years, and presents with mainly autonomic seizures.
3. Rolandic *focal* seizures occur in late childhood at a peak age of 7–8 years.

It is probably beneficial to analyse this further, as it is likely to aid our understanding of the disordered age-related maturational processes:

- In the first or early period (febrile seizures), the brain is vulnerable to seizures that are triggered by fever and mainly present with convulsions that are commonly generalised.
- The second or intermediate period (PS) consists of spontaneous seizures that are often prolonged for hours and present principally with autonomic and mainly emetic symptoms.
- The third or late period (rolandic seizures) consists of spontaneous focal sensorimotor seizures.

These three periods of clinical seizure susceptibility also have peculiar EEG accompaniments. The EEG is almost normal in the first period of febrile seizures, shows mainly posterior and multifocal spikes in the intermediate period of PS, and rolandic spikes in the late period of rolandic seizures.

All these indicate that the brain in early childhood has a low threshold to generalised convulsions provoked by fever, with a relatively silent EEG spike

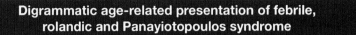

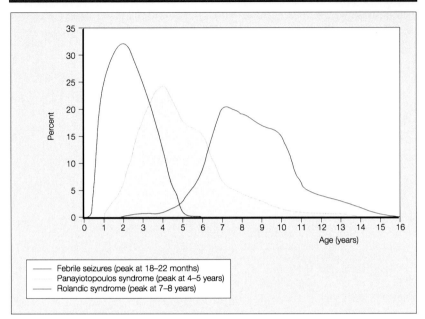

Figure 5.1 *Reproduced with permission from Panayiotopoulos (2002).*[90]

capacity. Subsequently, the autonomic system, and in particular the emetic centres, become vulnerable, the seizure discharges may be self-sustained and the cortex exhibits a diffuse multifocal epileptogenicity, which is unequally distributed and mainly affects the posterior regions. Finally, in the third period of late childhood, brain epileptogenicity shrinks to around the rolandic regions to produce the distinctive clinical and EEG manifestations of the rolandic syndrome.

These are incontrovertible facts about the developing brain that have not yet been explored, and we should also consider the neonatal and early infantile periods, because they have their own peculiarities, as indicated by the benign neonatal seizures that occur during the first few days of life, and the benign infantile focal seizures of Watanabe–Vigevano syndrome.

This point is exemplified by reports of children with neonatal seizures who later developed rolandic syndrome[160] or PS.[91] Maihara, *et al*[160] described a family with benign familial neonatal seizures in which two siblings later developed rolandic seizures and EEG CTSs. Lada, *et al*[91] reported an otherwise normal boy who first had benign neonatal seizures, and then two febrile seizures at the age of 18 months and 3 years. This was followed by a nocturnal autonomic seizure of PS with ictal vomiting and deviation of the eyes at 6 years of age; the EEG showed occipital paroxysms. I have also described a boy who, at 8 weeks, had three focal seizures of right-sided convulsions involving the face and upper limbs (benign infantile seizures of the Watanabe–Vigevano syndrome). Subsequent EEGs were normal and treatment was stopped at the age of 10 months. He was well until the age of 7 years when he started having rolandic seizures and later developed epilepsy with continuous spike-and-wave during sleep.[189] The brain MRI was normal (case 17.2 of Panayiotopoulos[1]).

Benign (Isolated) Focal Seizures of Adolescence

6

Benign (isolated) focal seizures of adolescence[161-168] constitute an idiopathic, short-lived and transient period of seizure susceptibility during the second decade of life. The seizures are single or occur in a cluster of up to five seizures over 36 hours, never to occur again.[168]

Considerations on classification

Benign (isolated) focal seizures of adolescence may be considered among 'conditions with epileptic seizures that do not require a diagnosis of epilepsy'.[2] They are not an ILAE-recognised syndrome.

Demographic data

The seizures start and end within the second decade of life with a peak onset at 13–15 years, and a 71.2% male preponderance. They may account for between 7.5%[169] and 22%[164,168] of patients who have simple focal seizures in the second decade of life. Around 200 cases have been described.[162,164,165,170,171]

Clinical manifestations

The syndrome manifests with a single seizure or a cluster of two to five focal seizures. There are no epileptic events before or after this limited seizure period, which lasts for no more than 36 hours. The physical and mental states of patients are normal.

Motor seizures, usually without jacksonian marching, and somatosensory seizures are the most common types. Visual, vertiginous and autonomic symptoms are reported in a fifth of cases. Temporal lobe seizures almost never occur, and most of the seizures are diurnal (87%).

The teenager is fully aware and can give a reliable account of the onset of the clinical manifestations (simple focal seizures) in the majority of episodes (88%). However, consciousness rarely remains intact throughout the whole event; the seizures usually evolve to impaired cognition and/or secondarily GTCSs, which occur in half the cases.

Diagnostic procedures

Laboratory tests and brain imaging are normal. The EEG may show some minor, non-specific abnormalities with no spikes or focal slowing. In a recent report, nine of 37 cases had functional spikes,[165] which is incompatible with this syndrome; these patients probably suffered from benign childhood focal seizures as described earlier.

Differential diagnosis

These patients are difficult to diagnose, because there are no specific features at onset to differentiate them from others with similar clinical manifestations, but with different aetiologies, such as symptomatic or cryptogenic focal epilepsies. My practice is to investigate all adolescents with onset of focal seizures using MRI and EEGs, which, if normal, would make the diagnosis of benign focal seizures of adolescence more likely. A definitive diagnosis cannot be made until the patient has been free of seizures for 1–5 years.[162,164]

Prognosis and management

The prognosis is excellent and no drug treatment is required because only one or a cluster of two to five focal seizures (which cannot be predicted) occur within 36 hours.

Management of Benign Childhood Focal Seizures

7

Short- and long-term treatment strategies of benign childhood focal seizures are empirical.[20] Current practice parameter guidelines for febrile seizures,[172,173] if appropriately modified, may be the basis for similar guidelines in benign childhood focal seizures.[20,90] Based on the risks and benefits of the effective therapies, continuous anti-epileptic medication is not recommended for children who have had only one or brief seizures. Most clinicians treat recurrent seizures with carbamazepine, but in exceptional cases this may worsen seizures. Lengthy convulsive seizures are a medical emergency; rectal or buccal benzodiazepam is prescribed for home administration. Recurrent and lengthy seizures create anxiety in parents and patients and, as such, appropriate education and emotional support should be provided.

Acute management of a child with prolonged seizures

Control of the seizure is paramount. On the rare occasions that the child is febrile, treatment of any fever and the underlying illness is also important.

Autonomic status epilepticus needs thorough evaluation for proper diagnosis and assessment of the neurological/autonomic state of the child. Aggressive treatment should be avoided because of the risk of iatrogenic complications, including cardiorespiratory arrest.[8,10]

Long-lasting convulsive seizures (>10 min) or convulsive status epilepticus (>30 min to hours), although rare, constitute a genuine paediatric emergency that demands appropriate and vigorous treatment.[189] Benzodiazepines, in intravenous, rectal or buccal preparations, are commonly used to terminate status epilepticus.

Early parental intervention is more effective than late emergency treatment.

Prophylactic anti-epileptic drug treatment of benign childhood focal seizures

Continuous AED treatment is not usually recommended. Although there are effective therapies that could prevent the occurrence of additional seizures, the potential adverse effects of such therapy are not commensurate with the benefit. The great majority of children with benign focal seizures do not need AED treatment even if they have lengthy seizures or more than two recurrences. The risks are small and the potential side effects of drugs appear to outweigh the benefits.

C.P. Panayiotopoulos, *Benign Childhood Focal Seizures and Related Epileptic Syndromes*, 47
© Springer-Verlag London Limited 2011

In patients with recurrent seizures and/or when parental anxiety associated with seizures is severe, small doses of AEDs may be effective in preventing a recurrence. There is no convincing evidence, however, that any therapy will alleviate the possibility of recurrences. In deciding management for a child with benign childhood focal seizures, the following should be considered:

- Most children have an excellent prognosis: about 10–30% of patients may have only a single seizure, and seizures may be infrequent (usually 2–10) in 60–70%. However, 10–20% of patients may have frequent seizures, which are sometimes resistant to treatment.
- Remission of benign childhood focal seizures is expected in all patients by the age of 15, or 16 years at the latest.
- The possibility of future epilepsy is a most unlikely event and probably not higher than that in the general population.
- There is no evidence that the long-term prognosis is worse in untreated children, although they may not be protected against seizure recurrences.
- Some children become frightened, even by simple focal seizures, and some parents are unable to cope with the possibility of another fit despite firm reassurances.
- Persistence and frequency of EEG functional spikes do not predict clinical severity, frequency or degree of liability to recurrent seizures.

Continuous prophylaxis consists of daily monotherapy using any AED that has proven efficacy in focal seizures and minimal adverse effects in children. The 2006 ILAE treatment guidelines found that 'no AED had level A or level B efficacy and effectiveness evidence as initial monotherapy' in rolandic epilepsy.[174] Of older AED most authorities prefer carbamazepine in USA[175] and valproate in Europe,[176] though these may have equivalent efficacy with phenobarbital, phenytoin and clonazepam;[17,84] carbamazepine may exaggerate seizures in a minority of children with BCSSS including PS[177] and valproate is associated with significant ADRs. Recently, sulthiame (available only in a few countries) has been revived as an excellent drug for the treatment of rolandic epilepsy with EEG normalisation[178–180] but this may be associated with cognitive abnormalities.[181] Recommended newer AED include levetiracetam,[76–78,182,183] oxcarbazepine[77] and gabapentin.[184] Lamotrigine is also used[175] though this drug have been associated in a few reports with seizure exacerbation and cognitive deterioration in rolandic epilepsy.[79–81,185]

Stopping medication

Strategies of withdrawing medication differ among experts, although all agree that there is no need to continue medication 1–3 years after the last seizure and certainly not after age 14 when most benign childhood focal seizures remit, or age 16, when they are practically non-existent. My practice is to start the gradual withdrawal of medication 2 years after the last seizure, making sure that the child does not have any minor seizures.

However, I do not adhere to fixed rules and may continue medication until age 13–15 years depending on the severity, frequency and age at onset of seizures. Thus, in a child with frequent, severe and difficult-to-control fits in early childhood, I would not stop medication if the child had a seizure-free period of 2 or 3 years by age 7. Conversely, for a child who had three or four nocturnal seizures at age 11 and 12, I would slowly discontinue medication after a 2-year seizure-free period. I advise very slow withdrawal, reducing the dose in monthly steps until complete discontinuation. I follow this procedure because I expect that any possible seizure recurrence during the process of very slow drug withdrawal would manifest with mild, brief and simple focal seizures with no secondarily GTCSs. In the case of phenobarbital and benzodiazepines, slow withdrawal of medication is mandatory to avoid risking withdrawal seizures.

Parental attitude and education

By Thalia Valeta

Benign childhood focal seizures, like febrile convulsions,[186] despite their excellent prognosis, are usually a dramatic experience for those parents who are young and inexperienced and often think that their child is dead or dying.[187]

In my study of parental attitude and reaction in benign childhood focal seizures and particularly PS,[187] the most common fears and expressions were:

> I thought he/she was dying, choking, asphyxiated, electrocuted, never to come around again.

> I thought he had a stroke.

> I was terrified, petrified.

> The doctor told me that because the seizure was longer than half an hour this may affect his brain and that time will tell.

> We sleep with our daughter in between us on a large bed, and we keep an eye on her as she enters and exits sleep.

The following are the most dominant points emerging from that study:[187]

- *Uncertainty of what this event was:* Most parents felt uncertain about what had happened and that they were not given sufficient information or reassurance; some were told that the child had not had a seizure. Initially, some children were diagnosed as having encephalitis, atypical migraine, fainting, gastroenteritis or motion sickness. Some parents of children with recurrent seizures found the correct diagnosis through their own research on the internet and in medical literature.
- *Anxiety about what caused the event:* This was often associated with a feeling of guilt – of parental acts directly associated with the event (child relatively unattended, preceding parental arguments, child involved in leisure activity that may have caused the attack), heredity or with

previous events in the child's development (birth, trauma, illness, family history of illness).

- *The effect of the seizure in the child's development:* 'Is this going to affect his or her brain?' The majority of parents were reassured that one brief seizure would not affect the child's development. However, some parents of children with lengthy seizures were left with the impression that because the seizure was prolonged, it may have had some adverse effect on the child and that only 'time will tell'.
- *Lack of advice regarding relapses:* No specific advice was provided about the possibility of relapses and what the parents should do if such a seizure recurred.

These results indicate that there is a need for supportive family management, education and specific instructions about emergency procedures for possible subsequent seizures. Demonstrations of first aid practices for seizures are necessary. Parents of young children should be given general information about benign childhood focal seizures and, in particular, PS, in which seizures may last for many hours, and which is compounded by physicians' uncertainty over diagnoses, management and prognosis. Parents who have watched their child during a fit need specific information and psychological support to overcome anxiety and panic. Anxiety may result in overprotection, which interferes with parent–child separation and independence.[187,188]

References

1. Panayiotopoulos CP. Benign childhood partial seizures and related epileptic syndromes. London: John Libbey & Co. Ltd, 1999.
2. Engel J, Jr. A proposed diagnostic scheme for people with epileptic seizures and with epilepsy: Report of the ILAE Task Force on Classification and Terminology. Epilepsia 2001;42:796–803.
3. Engel J, Jr. Report of the ILAE Classification Core Group. Epilepsia 2006;47:1558–68.
4. Ferrie CD, Grunewald RA. Panayiotopoulos syndrome: a common and benign childhood epilepsy. Lancet 2001;357:821–3.
5. Koutroumanidis M. Panayiotopoulos syndrome: a common benign but underdiagnosed and unexplored early childhood seizure syndrome. BMJ 2002;324:1228–9.
6. Covanis A. Panayiotopoulos syndrome: a benign childhood autonomic epilepsy frequently imitating encephalitis, syncope, migraine, sleep disorder, or gastroenteritis. Pediatrics 2006;118:e1237–43.
7. Koutroumanidis M. Panayiotopoulos syndrome: An important electroclinical example of benign childhood system epilepsy. Epilepsia 2007;48:1044–53.
8. Ferrie C, Caraballo R, Covanis A, Demirbilek V, Dervent A, Kivity S, et al. Panayiotopoulos syndrome: a consensus view. Dev Med Child Neurol 2006;48:236–40.
9. Caraballo R, Cersosimo R, Fejerman N. Panayiotopoulos syndrome: a prospective study of 192 patients. Epilepsia 2007;48:1054–61.
10. Ferrie CD, Caraballo R, Covanis A, Demirbilek V, Dervent A, Fejerman N, et al. Autonomic status epilepticus in Panayiotopoulos syndrome and other childhood and adult epilepsies: A consensus view. Epilepsia 2007;48:1165–72.
11. Martinovic Z. The new ILAE report on classification and evidence-based commentary on Panayiotopoulos syndrome and autonomic status epilepticus. Epilepsia 2007;48:1215–6.
12. Panayiotopoulos CP. The birth and evolution of the concept of Panayiotopoulos syndrome. Epilepsia 2007;48:1041–3.
13. Gibbs EL, Gillen HW, Gibbs FA. Disappearance and migration of epileptic foci in childhood. Am J Dis Child 1954;88:596–603.
14. Blume WT, Luders HO, Mizrahi E, Tassinari C, van Emde BW, Engel J, Jr. Glossary of descriptive terminology for ictal semiology: report of the ILAE task force on classification and terminology. Epilepsia 2001;42:1212–8.
15. Loiseau P, Beaussart M. The seizures of benign childhood epilepsy with rolandic paroxysmal discharges. Epilepsia 1973;14:381–9.
16. Loiseau P, Duche B. Benign rolandic epilepsy. Adv Neurol 1992;57:411–7.
17. Bouma PA, Bovenkerk AC, Westendorp RG, Brouwer OF. The course of benign partial epilepsy of childhood with centrotemporal spikes: a meta-analysis. Neurology 1997;48:430–7.
18. Beaussart M, Loiseau P, Roger H. The discovery of 'benign rolandic epilepsy'. In: Berkovic SF, Genton P, Hirsch E, Picard F, eds. Genetics of focal epilepsies, pp 3–6. London: John Libbey & Co. Ltd, 1999.
19. Fejerman N. Benign childhood epilepsy with centrotemporal spikes. In: Engel JJr, Pedley TA, eds. Philadelphia: Lippincott Williams & Wilkins, A Wolters Kluwer Business, 2008:2369–77.
20. Panayiotopoulos CP, Michael M, Sanders S, Valeta T, Koutroumanidis M. Benign childhood focal epilepsies: assessment of established and newly recognized syndromes. Brain 2008;131:2264–86.
21. Engel JJr, Fejerman N. Benign childhood epilepsy with centrotemporal spikes. http://www.ilae-epilepsy.org/Visitors/Centre/ctf/benign_child_centrotemp.html. Last accessed 15 November 2009.
22. Dalla Bernardina B, Sgro M, Fejerman N. Epilepsy with centro-temporal spikes and related syndromes. In: Roger J, Bureau M, Dravet C, Genton P, Tassinari CA, Wolf P, eds. Epileptic syndromes in infancy, childhood and adolescence. Fourth edition, pp 203–25. Montrouge, France: John Libbey Eurotext, 2005.
23. Covanis A, Lada C, Skiadas K. Children with rolandic spikes and ictus emeticus: rolandic epilepsy or Panayiotopoulos syndrome? Epileptic Disord 2003;5:139–43.
24. Fejerman N, Di Blasi AM. Status epilepticus of benign partial epilepsies in children: report of two cases. Epilepsia 1987;28:351–5.
25. Colamaria V, Sgro V, Caraballo R, Simeone M, Zullini E, Fontana E, et al. Status epilepticus in benign rolandic epilepsy manifesting as anterior operculum syndrome. Epilepsia 1991;32:329–34.
26. Deonna TW, Roulet E, Fontan D, Marcoz JP. Speech and oromotor deficits of epileptic origin in benign partial epilepsy of childhood with rolandic spikes (BPERS). Relationship to the acquired aphasia-epilepsy syndrome. Neuropediatrics 1993;24:83–7.

27. Fejerman N, Caraballo R, Tenembaum SN. [Atypical evolutions of benign partial epilepsy of infancy with centro- temporal spikes.] Rev Neurol 2000;31:389–96.

28. Fejerman N, Caraballo R, Tenembaum SN. Atypical evolutions of benign localization-related epilepsies in children: are they predictable? Epilepsia 2000;41:380–90.

29. Fejerman N, Caraballo RH, eds. Benign focal epilepsies in infancy, childhood and adolescence. John Libbey Eurotext, 2007.

30. Caraballo R, Fontana E, Michelizza B, Zullini B, Sgro V, Pajno-Ferrara F, et al. Carbamazepina, 'assenze atipiche', 'crisi atoniche', 'crisi atoniche' e stato di PO continua del sonno. Boll Lega It Epil 1989;66/67:379–81.

31. Parmeggiani L, Seri S, Bonanni P, Guerrini R. Electrophysiological characterization of spontaneous and carbamazepine-induced epileptic negative myoclonus in benign childhood epilepsy with centro-temporal spikes. Clin Neurophysiol 2004;115:50–8.

32. Vadlamudi L, Harvey AS, Connellan MM, Milne RL, Hopper JL, Scheffer IE, et al. Is benign rolandic epilepsy genetically determined? Ann Neurol 2004;56:129–32.

33. Neubauer BA, Fiedler B, Himmelein B, Kampfer F, Lassker U, Schwabe G, et al. Centrotemporal spikes in families with rolandic epilepsy: linkage to chromosome 15q14. Neurology 1998;51:1608–12.

34. Bray PF, Wiser WC. Evidence for a genetic etiology of temporal-central abnormalities in focal epilepsy. New Engl J Med 1964;271:926–33.

35. Strug LJ, Clarke T, Chiang T et al. Centrotemporal sharp wave EEG trait in rolandic epilepsy maps to Elongator Protein Complex 4 (ELP4). Eur J Hum Genet 2009;17:1171-81.

36. Panayiotopoulos CP. Benign childhood partial epilepsies: benign childhood seizure susceptibility syndromes. J Neurol Neurosurg Psychiatr 1993;56:2–5.

37. Gelisse P, Corda D, Raybaud C, Dravet C, Bureau M, Genton P. Abnormal neuroimaging in patients with benign epilepsy with centrotemporal spikes. Epilepsia 2003;44:372–8.

38. Lundberg S, Weis J, Eeg-Olofsson O, Raininko R. Hippocampal region asymmetry assessed by 1H-MRS in rolandic epilepsy. Epilepsia 2003;44:205–10.

39. Legarda S, Jayakar P, Duchowny M, Alvarez L, Resnick T. Benign rolandic epilepsy: high central and low central subgroups. Epilepsia 1994;35:1125–9.

40. De Marco P, Tassinari CA. Extreme somatosensory evoked potential (ESEP): an EEG sign forecasting the possible occurrence of seizures in children. Epilepsia 1981;22:569–75.

41. Tassinari CA, De Marco P, Plasmati R, Pantieri R, Blanco M, Michelucci R. Extreme somatosensory evoked potentials (ESEPs) elicited by tapping of hands or feet in children: a somatosensory cerebral evoked potentials study. Neurophysiol Clin 1988;18:123–8.

42. Minami T, Gondo K, Yanai S, Yamamoto T, Tasaki K, Ueda K. Rolandic discharges and somatosensory evoked potentials in benign childhood partial epilepsy: magnetoencephalographical study. Psychiatry Clin Neurosci 1995;49:S227–8.

43. Manganotti P, Miniussi C, Santorum E, Tinazzi M, Bonato C, Polo A, et al. Scalp topography and source analysis of interictal spontaneous spikes and evoked spikes by digital stimulation in benign rolandic epilepsy. Electroencephalogr Clin Neurophysiol 1998;107:18–26.

44. Manganotti P, Miniussi C, Santorum E, Tinazzi M, Bonato C, Marzi CA, et al. Influence of somatosensory input on paroxysmal activity in benign rolandic epilepsy with 'extreme somatosensory evoked potentials'. Brain 1998;121 Pt 4:647–58.

45. Fonseca LC, Tedrus GM. Somatosensory evoked spikes and epileptic seizures: a study of 385 cases. Clin Electroencephalogr 2000;31:71–5.

46. Kubota M, Takeshita K, Sakakihara Y, Yanagisawa M. Magnetoencephalographic study of giant somatosensory evoked responses in patients with rolandic epilepsy. J Child Neurol 2000;15:370–9.

47. Langill L, Wong PK. Tactile-evoked rolandic discharges: a benign finding? Epilepsia 2003;44:221–7.

48. Gregory DL, Wong PK. Clinical relevance of a dipole field in rolandic spikes. Epilepsia 1992;33:36–44.

49. Yoshinaga H, Sato M, Oka E, Ohtahara S. Spike dipole analysis using SEP dipole as a marker. Brain Topogr 1995;8:7–11.

50. Tsai ML, Hung KL. Topographic mapping and clinical analysis of benign childhood epilepsy with centrotemporal spikes. Brain Dev 1998;20:27–32.

51. Jung KY, Kim JM, Kim DW. Patterns of interictal spike propagation across the central sulcus in benign rolandic epilepsy. Clin Electroencephalogr 2003;34:153–7.

52. Minami T, Gondo K, Yamamoto T, Yanai S, Tasaki K, Ueda K. Magnetoencephalographic analysis of rolandic discharges in benign childhood epilepsy. Ann Neurol 1996;39:326–34.

53. Huiskamp G, van der MW, van Huffelen A, van Nieuwenhuizen O. High resolution spatio-temporal EEG-MEG analysis of rolandic spikes. J Clin Neurophysiol 2004;21:84–95.

54. Boor R, Jacobs J, Hinzmann A, Bauermann T, Scherg M, Boor S, et al. Combined spike-related functional MRI and multiple source analysis in the non-invasive spike localization of benign rolandic epilepsy. Clin Neurophysiol 2007;118:901–9.

55. Gibbs FA, Gibbs EL. Medical electroencephalography. Reading, MA: Addison-Wesley Publishing Co., 1967.

56. Petersen I, Eeg-Olofsson O. The development of the electroencephalogram in normal children from the age of 1 through 15 years. Non-paroxysmal activity. Neuropadiatrie 1971;2:247–304.
57. Cavazzuti GB, Cappella L, Nalin A. Longitudinal study of epileptiform EEG patterns in normal children. Epilepsia 1980;21:43–55.
58. Okubo Y, Matsuura M, Asai T, Asai K, Kato M, Kojima T, et al. Epileptiform EEG discharges in healthy children: prevalence, emotional and behavioral correlates, and genetic influences. Epilepsia 1994;35:832–41.
59. Panayiotopoulos CP, ed. A practical guide to childhood epilepsies. Oxford: Medicinae, 2006.
60. Beaumanoir A, Ballis T, Varfis G, Ansari K. Benign epilepsy of childhood with rolandic spikes. A clinical, electroencephalographic, and telencephalographic study. Epilepsia 1974;15:301–15.
61. Lerman P, Kivity S. Benign focal epilepsy of childhood. A follow-up study of 100 recovered patients. Arch Neurol 1975;32:261–4.
62. Blom S, Heijbel J. Benign epilepsy of children with centrotemporal EEG foci: a follow-up study in adulthood of patients initially studied as children. Epilepsia 1982;23:629–2.
63. Loiseau P, Pestre M, Dartigues JF, Commenges D, Barberger-Gateau C, Cohadon S. Long-term prognosis in two forms of childhood epilepsy: typical absence seizures and epilepsy with rolandic (centrotemporal) EEG foci. Ann Neurol 1983;13:642–8.
64. D'Alessandro P, Piccirilli M, Tiacci C, Ibba A, Maiotti M, Sciarma T, et al. Neuropsychological features of benign partial epilepsy in children. Ital J Neurol Sci 1990;11:265–9.
65. Piccirilli M, D'Alessandro P, Sciarma T, Cantoni C, Dioguardi MS, Giuglietti M, et al. Attention problems in epilepsy: possible significance of the epileptogenic focus. Epilepsia 1994;35:1091–6.
66. Baglietto MG, Battaglia FM, Nobili L, Tortorelli S, De Negri E, Calevo MG, et al. Neuropsychological disorders related to interictal epileptic discharges during sleep in benign epilepsy of childhood with centrotemporal or rolandic spikes. Dev Med Child Neurol 2001;43:407–12.
67. Nicolai J, Aldenkamp AP, Arends J, Weber JW, Vles JS. Cognitive and behavioral effects of nocturnal epileptiform discharges in children with benign childhood epilepsy with centrotemporal spikes. Epilepsy Behav 2006;8:56–70.
68. Kavros PM, Clarke T, Strug LJ, Halperin JM, Dorta NJ, Pal DK. Attention impairment in rolandic epilepsy: systematic review. Epilepsia 2008;49:1570–80.
69. Yung AW, Park YD, Cohen MJ, Garrison TN. Cognitive and behavioral problems in children with centrotemporal spikes. Pediatr Neurol 2000;23:391–5.
70. Pinton F, Ducot B, Motte J, Arbues AS, Barondiot C, Barthez MA, et al. Cognitive functions in children with benign childhood epilepsy with centrotemporal spikes (BECTS). Epileptic Disord 2006;8:11–23.
71. Giordani B, Caveney AF, Laughrin D, Huffman JL, Berent S, Sharma U, et al. Cognition and behavior in children with benign epilepsy with centrotemporal spikes (BECTS). Epilepsy Res 2006;70:89–94.
72. Liasis A, Bamiou DE, Boyd S, Towell A. Evidence for a neurophysiologic auditory deficit in children with benign epilepsy with centro-temporal spikes. J Neural Transm 2006;113:939–49.
73. Riva D, Vago C, Franceschetti S, Pantaleoni C, D'Arrigo S, Granata T, et al. Intellectual and language findings and their relationship to EEG characteristics in benign childhood epilepsy with centrotemporal spikes. Epilepsy Behav 2007; 10:278–85.
74. Al Twajri WA, Shevell MI. Atypical benign epilepsy of childhood with rolandic spikes: features of a subset requiring more than one medication for seizure control. J Child Neurol 2002;17:901–904.
75. Peters JM, Camfield CS, Camfield PR. Population study of benign rolandic epilepsy: Is treatment needed? Neurology 2001;57:537–539.
76. Verrotti A, Coppola G, Manco R, Ciambra G, Iannetti P, Grosso S, et al. Levetiracetam monotherapy for children and adolescents with benign rolandic seizures. Seizure 2007;16:271–5.
77. Coppola G, Franzoni E, Verrotti A, Garone C, Sarajlija J, Felicia OF, et al. Levetiracetam or oxcarbazepine as monotherapy in newly diagnosed benign epilepsy of childhood with centrotemporal spikes (BECTS): An open-label, parallel group trial. Brain Dev 2007;29:281–4.
78. Bello-Espinosa LE, Roberts SL. Levetiracetam for benign epilepsy of childhood with centrotemporal spikes-three cases. Seizure 2003;12:157–9.
79. Seidel WT, Mitchell WG. Cognitive and behavioral effects of carbamazepine in children: data from benign rolandic epilepsy. J Child Neurol 1999;14:716–23.
80. Catania S, Cross H, de Sousa C, Boyd S. Paradoxic reaction to lamotrigine in a child with benign focal epilepsy of childhood with centrotemporal spikes. Epilepsia 1999;40:1657–60.
81. Cerminara C, Montanaro ML, Curatolo P, Seri S. Lamotrigine-induced seizure aggravation and negative myoclonus in idiopathic rolandic epilepsy. Neurology 2004;63:373–5.
82. Panayiotopoulos CP. Inhibitory effect of central vision on occipital lobe seizures. Neurology 1981;31:1330–3.
83. Panayiotopoulos CP. Vomiting as an ictal manifestation of epileptic seizures and syndromes. J Neurol Neurosurg Psychiatr 1988;51:1448–51.
84. Ferrie CD, Beaumanoir A, Guerrini R, Kivity S, Vigevano F, Takaishi Y, et al. Early-onset benign occipital seizure susceptibility syndrome. Epilepsia 1997;38:285–93.

85. Oguni H, Hayashi K, Imai K, Hirano Y, Mutoh A, Osawa M. Study on the early-onset variant of benign childhood epilepsy with occipital paroxysms otherwise described as early-onset benign occipital seizure susceptibility syndrome. Epilepsia 1999;40:1020–30.

86. Kivity S, Ephraim T, Weitz R, Tamir A. Childhood epilepsy with occipital paroxysms: clinical variants in 134 patients. Epilepsia 2000;41:1522–3.

87. Caraballo R, Cersosimo R, Medina C, Fejerman N. Panayiotopoulos-type benign childhood occipital epilepsy: a prospective study. Neurology 2000;55:1096–100.

88. Yalcin AD, Toydemir HE, Celebi LG, Forta H. Panayiotopoulos syndrome with coincidental brain lesions. Epileptic Disord 2009;11:270–6.

89. Dura-Trave T, Yoldi-Petri ME, Gallinas-Victoriano F. Panayiotopoulos syndrome: epidemiological and clinical characteristics and outcome. Eur J Neurol 2008;15:336–41.

90. Panayiotopoulos CP. Panayiotopoulos syndrome: A common and benign childhood epileptic syndrome. London: John Libbey & Co. Ltd, 2002.

91. Lada C, Skiadas K, Theodorou V, Covanis A. A study of 43 patients with Panayiotopoulos syndrome: A common and benign childhood seizure suceptibility. Epilepsia 2003;44:81–8.

92. Ohtsu M, Oguni H, Hayashi K, Funatsuka M, Imai K, Osawa M. EEG in children with early-onset benign occipital seizure susceptibility syndrome: Panayiotopoulos syndrome. Epilepsia 2003;44:435–42.

93. Demirbilek V, Dervent A. Panayiotopoulos syndrome: video-EEG illustration of a typical seizure. Epileptic Disord 2004;6:121–4.

94. Sanders S, Rowlinson S, Manidakis I, Ferrie CD, Koutroumanidis M. The contribution of the EEG technologists in the diagnosis of Panayiotopoulos syndrome (susceptibility to early onset benign childhood autonomic seizures). Seizure 2004;13:565–73.

95. Covanis A, Ferrie CD, Koutroumanidis M, Oguni H, Panayiotopoulos CP. Panayiotopoulos syndrome and Gastaut type idiopathic childhood occipital epilepsy. In: Roger J, Bureau M, Dravet C, Genton P, Tassinari CA, Wolf P, eds. Epileptic syndromes in infancy, childhood and adolescence. Fourth edition with video, pp 227–53. Montrouge, France: John Libbey Eurotext, 2005.

96. Tedrus GM, Fonseca LC. Autonomic seizures and autonomic status epilepticus in early onset benign childhood occipital epilepsy (Panayiotopoulos syndrome). Arq Neuropsiquiatr 2006;64:723–26.

97. Ohtsu M, Oguni H, Imai K, Funatsuka M, Osawa M. Early-onset form of benign childhood epilepsy with centro-temporal EEG foci - a different nosological perspective from panayiotopoulos syndrome. Neuropediatrics 2008;39:14–9.

98. Panayiotopoulos CP. Benign childhood epilepsy with occipital paroxysms: a 15-year prospective study. Ann Neurol 1989;26:51–6.

99. Panayiotopoulos CP. Extraoccipital benign childhood partial seizures with ictal vomiting and excellent prognosis. J Neurol Neurosurg Psychiatry 1999;66:82–5.

100. Verrotti A, Salladini C, Trotta D, di Corcia G, Chiarelli F. Ictal cardiorespiratory arrest in Panayiotopoulos syndrome. Neurology 2005;64:1816–7.

101. Panayiotopoulos CP. Autonomic seizures and autonomic status epilepticus peculiar to childhood: diagnosis and management. Epilepsy Behav 2004;5:286–95.

102. Schnipper JL, Kapoor WN. Diagnostic evaluation and management of patients with syncope. Med Clin North Am 2001;85:423–56,xi.

103. Lempert T. Recognizing syncope: pitfalls and surprises. J R Soc Med 1996;89:372–5.

104. Livingston JH, Cross JH, McLellan A, Birch R, Zuberi SM. A Novel Inherited Mutation in the Voltage Sensor Region of SCN1A Is Associated With Panayiotopoulos Syndrome in Siblings and Generalized Epilepsy With Febrile Seizures Plus. J Child Neurol 2009;24:503–8.

105. Grosso S, Orrico A, Galli S, Di Bartolo R, Sorrentino V, Balestri P. SCN1A mutation associated with atypical Panayiotopoulos syndrome. Neurology 2007;69:609–11.

106. Burgess RC. Autonomic signs associated with seizures. In: Luders HO, Noachtar S, eds. Epileptic seizures. Pathophysiology and clinical semiology, pp 631–41. New York: Churchill Livingstone, 2000.

107. Baumgartner C, Lurger S, Leutmezer F. Autonomic symptoms during epileptic seizures. Epileptic Disord 2001;3:103–16.

108. Luders HO, Noachtar S, Burgess RC. Semiologic classification of epileptic seizures. In: Luders HO, Noachtar S, eds. Epileptic seizures. Pathophysiology and clinical semiology, pp 263–285. New York: Churchill Livingstone, 2000.

109. Schauble B, Britton JW, Mullan BP, Watson J, Sharbrough FW, Marsh WR. Ictal vomiting in association with left temporal lobe seizures in a left hemisphere language-dominant patient. Epilepsia 2002;43:1432–5.

110. Koutroumanidis M. Ictal vomiting in association with left temporal lobe seizures in a left hemisphere language-dominant patient. Epilepsia 2003;44:1259.

111. Li BU, Issenman RM, Sarna SK. Consensus statement – 2nd International Scientific Symposium on CVS. The Faculty of the 2nd International Scientific Symposium on Cyclic Vomiting Syndrome. Dig Dis Sci 1999;44 Suppl 8:9S–11S.

112. Yoshinaga H, Koutroumanidis M, Shirasawa A, Kikumoto K, Ohtsuka Y, Oka E. Dipole analysis in panayiotopoulos syndrome. Brain Dev 2005;27:46–52.

113. Yoshinaga H, Koutroumanidis M, Kobayashi K, Shirasawa A, Kikumoto K, Inoue T, et al. EEG dipole characteristics in Panayiotopoulos syndrome. Epilepsia 2006;47:781–7.

114. Koutroumanidis M, Rowlinson S, Sanders S. Recurrent autonomic status epilepticus in Panayiotopoulos syndrome: video/EEG studies. Epilepsy Behav 2005;7:543–7.

115. Iannetti P, Spalice A, Rocchi V, Verrotti A. Diffuse onset of ictal electroencephalography in a typical case of panayiotopoulos syndrome and review of the literature. J Child Neurol 2009;24:472–6.

116. Beaumanoir A. Semiology of occipital seizures in infants and children. In: Andermann F, Beaumanoir A, Mira L, Roger J, Tassinari CA, eds. Occipital seizures and epilepsies in children, pp 71–86. London: John Libbey and Co. Ltd, 1993.

117. Kanazawa O, Tohyama J, Akasaka N, Kamimura T. A magnetoencephalographic study of patients with Panayiotopoulos syndrome. Epilepsia 2005;46:1106–13.

118. Saito N, Kanazawa O, Tohyama J et al. Brain Maturation-Related Spike Localization in Panayiotopoulos Syndrome: Magnetoencephalographic Study. Pediatr Neurol 2008;38:104–10.

119. Saitoh N, Kanazawa O, Toyama J, Akasaka N, Kamimura T. Magnetoencephalographic findings of Panayiotopoulos syndrome with frontal epileptic discharges. Pediatr Neurol 2007;36:190–194.

120. Hirano Y, Oguni H, Funatsuka M, Imai K, Osawa M. Neurobehavioral abnormalities may correlate with increased seizure burden in children with Panayiotopoulos syndrome. Pediatr Neurol 2009;40:443–8.

121. Caraballo RH, Astorino F, Cersosimo R, Soprano AM, Fejerman N. Atypical evolution in childhood epilepsy with occipital paroxysms (Panayiotopoulos type). Epileptic Disord 2001;3:157–62.

122. Ferrie CD, Koutroumanidis M, Rowlinson S, Sanders S, Panayiotopoulos CP. Atypical evolution of Panayiotopoulos syndrome: a case report [published with video- sequences.] Epileptic Disord 2002;4:35–42.

123. Germano E, Gagliano A, Magazu A, Sferro C, Calarese T, Mannarino E, et al. Benign childhood epilepsy with occipital paroxysms: Neuropsychological findings. Epilepsy Res 2005;64:137–50.

124. Camfield P, Camfield C. Sudden unexpected death in people with epilepsy: a pediatric perspective. Semin Pediatr Neurol 2005;12:10–4.

125. Gastaut H. A new type of epilepsy: benign partial epilepsy of childhood with occipital spike-waves. Clin Electroencephalogr 1982;13:13–22.

126. Gastaut H, Zifkin BG. Benign epilepsy of childhood with occipital spike and wave complexes. In: Andermann F, Lugaresi E, eds. Migraine and epilepsy, pp 47–81. Boston: Butterworths, 1987.

127. Gastaut H, Roger J, Bureau M. Benign epilepsy of childhood with occipital paroxysms. Up-date. In: Roger J, Bureau M, Dravet C, Dreifuss FE, Perret A, Wolf P, eds. Epileptic syndromes in infancy, childhood and adolescence. Second edition, pp 201–17. London: John Libbey & Co. Ltd, 1992.

128. Panayiotopoulos CP. Idiopathic childhood occipital epilepsies. In: Roger J, Bureau M, Dravet C, Genton P, Tassinari CA, Wolf P, eds. Epileptic syndromes in infancy, childhood and adolescence. Third edition, pp 203–227. London: John Libbey & Co Ltd, 2002.

129. Caraballo RH, Koutroumanidis M, Panayiotopoulos CP, Fejerman N. Idiopathich childhood occipital epilepsy of Gastaut. J Child Neurol 2009;24:1536–1542.

130. Commission on Classification and Terminology of the International League Against Epilepsy. Proposal for revised classification of epilepsies and epileptic syndromes. Epilepsia 1989;30:389–99.

131. Panayiotopoulos CP. Elementary visual hallucinations, blindness, and headache in idiopathic occipital epilepsy: differentiation from migraine. J Neurol Neurosurg Psychiatry 1999;66:536–40.

132. Nagendran K, Prior PF, Rossiter MA. Benign occipital epilepsy of childhood: a family study. J R Soc Med 1990;83:804–5.

133. Panayiotopoulos CP. Visual phenomena and headache in occipital epilepsy: a review, a systematic study and differentiation from migraine. Epileptic Disord 1999;1:205–16.

134. Panayiotopoulos CP. Occipital spikes, occipital paroxysms and other electroencephalographic findings in children with benign childhood occipital seizures . Occipital spikes in normal children and those without seizures. In: Panayiotopoulos CP, ed. Benign childhood partial seizures and related epileptic syndromes, pp 173–202. London: John Libbey & Co. Ltd, 1999.

135. Gibbs FA, Gibbs EL. Atlas of electroencephalography, Volume 2. Epilepsy, pp 214–290. Reading, MA: Addison-Wesley, 1952.

136. Kellaway P. The incidence, significance and natural history of spike foci in children. In: Henry CE, ed. Current clinical neurophysiology. Update on EEG and evoked potentials, pp 151–175. New York: Elsevier/North Holland, 1980.

137. Aso K, Watanabe K, Negoro T, Takaesu E, Furune A, Takahashi I, et al. Visual seizures in children. Epilepsy Res 1987;1:246–53.

138. De Romanis F, Feliciani M, Cerbo R. Migraine and other clinical syndromes in children affected by EEG occipital spike-wave complexes. Funct Neurol 1988;3:187–203.

139. De Romanis F, Buzzi MG, Cerbo R, Feliciani M, Assenza S, Agnoli A. Migraine and epilepsy with infantile onset and electroencephalographic findings of occipital spike-wave complexes. Headache 1991;31:378–83.

140. De Romanis F, Buzzi MG, Assenza S, Brusa L, Cerbo R. Basilar migraine with electroencephalographic findings of occipital spike-wave complexes: a long-term study in seven children. Cephalalgia 1993;13:192–6;discussion 150.

141. Beaumanoir A. An EEG contribution to the study of migraine and of the association between migraine and epilepsy in childhood. In: Andermann F, Beaumanoir A, Mira L, Roger J, Tassinari CA, eds. Occipital seizures and epilepsy in children, pp 101–10. London: John Libbey & company Ltd, 1993.

142. Panayiotopoulos CP. Basilar migraine: a review. In: Panayiotopoulos CP, ed. Benign childhood partial seizures and related epileptic syndromes, pp 303–8. London: John Libbey & Co. Ltd, 1999.

143. Gobbi G, Bertani G, Italian Working Group on Coeliac Disease and Epilepsy. Coeliac disease and epilepsy. In: Gobbi G, Andermann F, Naccarato S, Banchini G, eds. Epilepsy and other neurological disorders in coeliac disease, pp 65–79. London: John Libbey & Co. Ltd, 1997.

144. Taylor I, Berkovic SF, Kivity S, Scheffer IE. Benign occipital epilepsies of childhood: clinical features and genetics. Brain 2008;131:2287-94.

145. Tenembaum S, Deonna T, Fejerman N, Medina C, Ingvar-Maeder M, Gubser-Mercati D. Continuous spike-waves and dementia in childhood epilepsy with occipital paroxysms. J Epilepsy 1997;10:139–45.

146. Caraballo RH, Cersosimo RO, Fejerman N. Late-onset, "Gastaut type", childhood occipital epilepsy: an unusual evolution. Epileptic Disord 2005;7:341–6.

147. Gulgonen S, Demirbilek V, Korkmaz B, Dervent A, Townes BD. Neuropsychological functions in idiopathic occipital lobe epilepsy. Epilepsia 2000;41:405–11.

148. Dalla Bernardina B, Colamaria V, Chiamenti C, Capovilla G, Trevisan E, Tassinari CA. Benign partial epilepsy with affective symptoms ('benign psychomotor epilepsy'). In: Roger J, Bureau M, Dravet C, Dreifuss FE, Perret A, Wolf P, eds. Epileptic syndromes in infancy, childhood and adolescence. Second edition, pp 219–23. London: John Libbey & Co. Ltd, 1992.

149. Tassinari CA, De Marco P. Benign partial epilepsy with extreme somato-sensory evoked potentials. In: Roger J, Bureau M, Dravet C, Dreifuss FE, Wolf P, Perret A, eds. Epileptic syndromes in infancy, childhood and adolescense. Second edition, pp 225–9. London: John Libbey & Co. Ltd, 1992.

150. Negrin P, De Marco P. Parietal focal spikes evoked by tactile somatotopic stimulation in sixty non-epileptic children: the nocturnal sleep and clinical and EEG evolution. Electroencephalogr Clin Neurophysiol 1977;43:312–6.

151. Beaumanoir A, Nahory A. [Benign partial epilepsies: 11 cases of frontal partial epilepsy with favorable prognosis.] Rev Electroencephalogr Neurophysiol Clin 1983;13:207–11.

152. Martin-Santidrian MA, Garaizar C, Prats-Vinas JM. [Frontal lobe epilepsy in infancy: is there a benign partial frontal lobe epilepsy?] Rev Neurol 1998;26:919–23.

153. Bagdorf R, Lee SI. Midline spikes: is it another benign EEG pattern of childhood? Epilepsia 1993;34:271–4.

154. Kutluay E, Passaro EA, Gomez-Hassan D, Beydoun A. Seizure semiology and neuroimaging findings in patients with midline spikes. Epilepsia 2001;42:1563–8.

155. Sanders S, Rowlinson S, Koutroumanidis M, Ferrie CD, Panayiotopoulos CP. Midline spikes in children and clinical correlations. Epilepsia 2002;43:1436–9.

156. Bureau M, Cokar O, Maton B, Genton P, Dravet C. Sleep-related, low voltage Rolandic and vertex spikes: an EEG marker of benignity in infancy-onset focal epilepsies. Epileptic Disord 2002;4:15–22.

157. Capovilla G, Beccaria F. Benign partial epilepsy in infancy and early childhood with vertex spikes and waves during sleep: a new epileptic form. Brain Dev 2000;22:93–8.

158. Capovilla G, Beccaria F, Montagnini A. 'Benign focal epilepsy in infancy with vertex spikes and waves during sleep'. Delineation of the syndrome and recalling as 'benign infantile focal epilepsy with midline spikes and waves during sleep' (BIMSE). Brain Dev 2006;28:85–91.

159. Capovilla G, Beccaria F. Other phenotypes of BCSSS. In: Panayiotopoulos CP, ed. Atlas of epilepsies. London: Springer, 2010 (in press).

160. Maihara T, Tsuji M, Higuchi Y, Hattori H. Benign familial neonatal convulsions followed by benign epilepsy with centrotemporal spikes in two siblings. Epilepsia 1999;40:110–3.

161. Loiseau P, Orgogozo JM. An unrecognized syndrome of benign focal epileptic seizures in teenagers? Lancet 1978;2:1070–1.

162. Loiseau P, Louiset P. Benign partial seizures of adolescence. In: Roger J, Bureau M, Dravet C, Dreifuss FE, Perret A, Wolf P, eds. Epileptic syndromes in infancy, childhood and adolescence, pp 343–5. London: John Libbey & Co. Ltd, 1992.

163. Caraballo R, Galicchio S, Granana N, Cersosimo R, Fejerman N. [Benign partial convulsions in adolescence.] Rev Neurol 1999;28:669–71.

164. King MA, Newton MR, Berkovic SF. Benign partial seizures of adolescence. Epilepsia 1999;40:1244–7.

165. Capovilla G, Gambardella A, Romeo A, Beccaria F, Montagnini A, Labate A, et al. Benign partial epilepsies of adolescence: a report of 37 new cases. Epilepsia 2001;42:1549–52.

166. Caraballo RH, Cersosimo RO, Fejerman N. Benign focal seizures of adolescence: a prospective study. Epilepsia 2004;45:1600–3.

167. Panayiotopoulos CP. Benign childhood focal seizures and related epileptic syndromes. In: Panayiotopoulos CP, ed. The epilepsies: seizures, syndromes and management, pp 223–69. Oxford: Bladon Medical Publishing, 2005.
168. Loiseau P, Jallon P, Wolf P. Isolated partial seizures of adolescence. In: Roger J, Bureau M, Dravet C, Genton P, Tassinari CA, Wolf P, eds. Epileptic syndromes in infancy, childhood and adolescence. Fourth edition, pp 359–62. Montrouge: John Libbey Eurotext, 2005.
169. Panayiotopoulos CP. Benign partial seizures of adolescence. In: Wallace S, ed. Epilepsy in children, pp 377–8. London: Chapman & Hall, 1996.
170. Mauri JA, Iniguez C, Jerico I, Morales F. Benign partial seizures of adolescence. Epilepsia 1996;37 Suppl 4:102.
171. Jallon P, Loiseau J, Loiseau P, de Zelicourt M, Motte J, Vallee L, et al. The risk of recurrence after a first unprovoked seizure in adolescence. Epilepsia 1999;40 Suppl 7:87–8.
172. American Academy of Pediatrics. Practice parameter: long-term treatment of the child with simple febrile seizures. American Academy of Pediatrics. Committee on Quality Improvement, Subcommittee on Febrile Seizures. Pediatrics 1999:103 Pt 1:1307–9.
173. Baumann RJ. Technical report: treatment of the child with simple febrile seizures. Pediatrics 1999;103:e86.
174. Glauser T, Ben-Menachem E, Bourgeois B et al. ILAE treatment guidelines: evidence-based analysis of antiepileptic drug efficacy and effectiveness as initial monotherapy for epileptic seizures and syndromes. Epilepsia 2006;47:1094–120.
175. Wheless JW, Clarke DF, Carpenter D. Treatment of pediatric epilepsy: expert opinion, 2005. J Child Neurol 2005;20 Suppl 1:S1–56.
176. Wheless JW, Clarke DF, Arzimanoglou A, Carpenter D. Treatment of pediatric epilepsy: European expert opinion, 2007. Epileptic Disord 2007;9:353–412.
177. Kikumoto K, Yoshinaga H, Oka M, Ito M, Endoh F, Akiyama T, et al. EEG and seizure exacerbation induced by carbamazepine in Panayiotopoulos syndrome. Epileptic Disord 2006;8:53–6.
178. Engler F, Maeder-Ingvar M, Roulet E, Deonna T. Treatment with Sulthiame (Ospolot) in benign partial epilepsy of childhood and related syndromes: an open clinical and EEG study. Neuropediatrics, 2003;34:105–9.
179. Rating D, Wolf C, Bast T. Sulthiame as monotherapy in children with benign childhood epilepsy with centrotemporal spikes: a 6-month randomized, double-blind, placebo-controlled study. Sulthiame Study Group. Epilepsia 2000;41:1284–8.
180. Bast T, Volp A, Wolf C, Rating D. The influence of sulthiame on EEG in children with benign childhood epilepsy with centrotemporal spikes (BECTS). Epilepsia 2003;44:215–20.
181. Wirrell E, Sherman EM, Vanmastrigt R, Hamiwka L. Deterioration in cognitive function in children with benign epilepsy of childhood with central temporal spikes treated with sulthiame. J Child Neurol 2008;23:14–21.
182. Kossoff EH, Los JG, Boatman DF. A pilot study transitioning children onto levetiracetam monotherapy to improve language dysfunction associated with benign rolandic epilepsy. Epilepsy Behav 2007;11:514–7.
183. Garcia C, Rubio G. Efficacy and safety of levetiracetam in the treatment of Panayiotopoulos syndrome. Epilepsy Res 2009;85:318–20.
184. Bourgeois BF. Drug treatment of benign focal epilepsies of childhood. Epilepsia 2000;41:1057–8.
185. Battaglia D, Iuvone L, Stefanini MC et al. Reversible aphasic disorder induced by lamotrigine in atypical benign childhood epilepsy. Epileptic Disord 2001;3:217–22.
186. Balslev T. Parental reactions to a child's first febrile convulsion. A follow-up investigation. Acta Paediatr Scand 1991;80:466–9.
187. Valeta T. Parental attitude, reaction and education in benign childhood focal seizures. In: Panayiotopoulos CP, ed. The epilepsies: seizures, syndromes and management, pp 258–61. Oxford: Bladon Medical Publishing, 2005.
188. Valeta T, Sogawa Y, Moshe SL. Impact of focal seizures on patients and family. In: Panayiotopoulos CP, Benbadis S, Sisodiya S, eds. Volume 5: Focal epilepsies: seizures, syndromes and management. Oxford: Medicinae, 2008:230–8.
189. Panayiotopoulos CP. Clinical guide to epileptic syndromes and their treatment. Revised second edition. London: Springer, 2010.
190. Berg AT, Berkovic SF, Brodie MJ, Buchhalter J, Cross HJ, Van Emde Boas W et al. Revised terminology and concepts for organization of seizures and epilepsies: Report of the ILAE Commission on Classification and Terminology, 2005-2009. Epilepsia 2010; 51:676-685.
191. Ferrie CD, Livingston JH. Panayiotopoulos syndrome: learning lessons from atypical cases. Epileptic Disord 2010; 12(1):92-94.
192. Yalcin AD, Toydemir HE, Celebi LG, Forta H. Panayiotopoulos syndrome with coincidental brain lesions. Epileptic Disord 2009; 11(3):270-276.
193. Specchio N, Trivisano M, Balestri M, Cappelletti S, Di Ciommo V, Gentile S et al. Panayiotopoulos syndrome: A Clinical, EEG and Neuropsychological Study of 93 Consecutive Patients. Epilepsia (in press) 2010.

Index

Page numbers followed by **b** indicate boxes, page numbers followed by **f** indicate figures, and page numbers followed by **t** indicate tables.